ACKNOWLEDGEMENTS

I thank my wife Lena (Yelena) for her support and patience while I was working on this book. Most important, my thanks for help in arranging the publication.

I thank my friend Vincent Daddiego for his contribution and helpful review and comments.

My thanks and gratitude to the doctor (The Prince) for taking care of Elizabeth. Without him, this book would not be possible. I have withheld his real name for obvious reasons. He will, however, surely recognize himself.

In Honor and Memory of my wife
Elizabeth Sonnenberg who stood by me
for almost forty years.

HOW I KEPT

ELIZABETH

ALIVE

By Sven Sonnenberg

"You have done a splendid job of keeping
Elizabeth alive," the doctor said to me.
This book is devoted to all those countless men
who need to support the woman they love as
she goes through the ordeal of cancer.

CONTENTS

PREFACE

If you have this book in your hands, you are interested in the subject matter for serious reasons. It is possible, that one of your loved ones is in need of help or you, for yourself, decided to seek knowledge beyond what your doctor told you. It is especially important for those who are unfortunate to be stricken by cancer to have a close family member or a close friend take up the search for help. To educate himself and then try to get the ill spouse or friend to listen and cooperate in searching for a cure, or at least to augment and aid in whatever "official" medicine orders, if that is the decision—to follow the beaten path.

This account was originally written almost 14 years ago. I, however, recently learned of and followed the case of my neighbor who contracted breast cancer. Not much has changed over the years. My neighbor is just finishing, at this writing, the standard course of treatment at a leading institution, the so-called "Comprehensive Cancer Treatment Center" attached to a leading University Center. That center claims to be in the forefront of cancer treatment, research, and teaching. This neighbor went through the standard approach — surgery (lumpectomy), chemotherapy and then radiation. The cancer was a rather early stage, without metastases. My observation was that the chemo compounds used in this case were the same as I remember having been used 14 years ago, with no modification, even with all the auxiliary compounds, like easing nausea. The only change was guarding against infections this time, by lavish application of white cell support. In case of metastasis disease, the routines remained the same. The statistics today of survival in metastasis and recurrences in simple cases remain virtually the same as 14 years ago. The claim is that the death rate for breast cancer has declined by 2.2% per year for some groups of women, whereas for others it remained the same. One has to remember that since 2002 there was a sharp decline in the use of HRT (Hormone Replacement Therapy) after the findings, because it caused an increase in breast cancer. That caused a decline in breast cancer cases since 2002 and says very little about the efficacy of treatments, which virtually have not changed. So, one is hard pressed to assume that any progress in treatment has made a difference.

However, in some cancer cases the picture has changed for the better. In addition, progress has been made in new approaches in mainstream medicine. Unfortunately, these new approaches have not yet reached the clinical setting. The oncologist in the typical comprehensive center will still reach for Fluorouracil, Adriamycin, **Doxorubicin**, cyclophosphamide and paclitaxel et cetera, et cetera and all the other poisons, which have this shotgun approach to kill everything in sight and in many cases causing havoc in the body with often disastrous consequences further down the line in a setting of prolonged application. These include, but are not limited to heart failure, peripheral neuropathy, and gastrointestinal problems, while having only achieved short-term success. How short or long? No one can predict. Some may say okay, three to five or even ten years is not such a bad deal. Well, again I have an old neighbor who was found to have a cancerous polyp in his colon. He would have lived out his years if undisturbed, he was past 80 years old and died promptly after the second application of a harsh chemo. The doctor who was asked to stop it when bad side effects occurred did not, and that amounted to killing by chemo. That doctor was much unperturbed, as if it was a routine event.

It is therefore important to make one's own judgments, carry them through and most important: to seek out what is now available, but not yet practiced by the routine oncologist and to get to the place where it is. That takes time and effort and the person who is ill is not well-suited to do this. A dedicated friend or spouse must do it. The often-unfortunate situation is a lack of cooperation by the patient. My friend's wife became sick and refused to do anything of the program he asked me to send to him, and stuck strictly to what the doctor ordered and was dead in 6 months.

THIS BOOK IS NOT INTENDED TO HARSHLY
CRITICIZE OR CONDEMN THE MAINSTREAM
OFFICIAL MEDICINE SYSTEM. IT IS A CALL TO
BE COGNIZANT OF ITS WEAKNESSES AND
SHORTCOMINGS, TO MAKE THE PATIENT
AND ADVOCATE AWARE OF IT TO BETTER
HELP LOVED RELATIVES OR FRIENDS AND
HELP THEM THINK ABOUT AND CHOOSE A
COURSE OF ACTION.

INTRODUCTION

This narrative grew with the unfolding of events. My lifelong training in research and development required unswerving adherence to a strict observation of facts, lest my organization face failure. Given that, I must conclude that the description of ensuing events could not be closer to reality.

This is a cry to warn others to be alert and not allow being led wantonly down the "protocol" path without a fight. I have refrained for some time from any attempt at publishing this material. I hoped that I could work within the medical establishment to be of help that way, to improve the situation for those who would be forced onto a similar path by cruel fate. I suppressed my urges, reasoning that maybe by working from within I could do some good in a constructive way and forgo all my misgivings about the community of health practitioners. This was not to be. Therefore, I feel free and unbound by any constraints to go ahead and find someone who will be interested and will publish this account. I will paraphrase here the earthy Lyndon Johnson.

"No, don't fire that guy. I prefer him to be in the tent pissing out rather than outside pissing in."

I was left outside. Events unfolded to give me additional insights into this segment of our society – the medical establishment, on which we all so heavily rely for our welfare and that of our families. We run to it for help in the darkest hours of our lives!

Before I left for Los Angeles, the doctor I call the Prince (Dr. Hope who was the principal doctor) called me to say good luck and to contact him on my return.

"You have done a splendid job of keeping Elizabeth alive. I will have some work for you at the Clinic when you return," he said.

I notified him of my return and said I was ready any time. His response to my e-mail was:

"I hope everything went well in California. I would like to make use of your many talents in helping our breast cancer research effort become better organized..."

I was very grateful. This was what I could do in my life, empty now without Elizabeth. I had put an enormous effort into study, research, and practical steps trying to save Elizabeth. I was told I produced stunning results. It was not good enough! The sense of failure was overwhelming despite all the reassurances I received from every corner about my efforts. I was just not used to losing battles and the Prince's offer was a way for me to compensate, in a way, for my failure. Maybe I could win some small victories against that scourge that took the essence of my life away.

I waited five months for the Prince to put me to work. I reminded him by mail, and spoke to him verbally. He sounded so convincing that I could not doubt his sincerity. What happened, why he never came through, is pure guesswork. I will not speculate. The fact remains that this was my only opening to do this kind of work because he had known me for such a long time and had observed me in action. Anybody else in that establishment would laugh an engineer out of the interview room.

Almost coincidentally while finishing these words the call came from the Prince. "I need you badly, come in and see me," he said. I worked for a few days doing all kinds of chores with enthusiasm, hoping that I could slowly work myself into the organization and make some difference. A week later, the Prince said, "I have gotten objections to your presence around the office from my people"

"Doc, aren,t you the director?"

"Yes, but I cannot ignore their arguments. We will have to work after hours and on weekends. You can take some things to do at home."

I completed a number of assignments for him and was hoping that when his new Clinic was established my work would become steadier and its importance would increase. This hope was augmented by the fact that he often expressed satisfaction with my work. I patiently weathered long waits for his attention and non-responses to my initiatives. Finally, the Clinic started operations and I started working half-days. That ended one day with the Prince asking me to page him before I came in, he again had objection from his organization to keep an engineer. He never responded to my page or follow up e-mail, has not even checked to see if I am still alive. I have decided then to go ahead with my idea to place this account with someone. *I also decided not to include any information or expressions from anyone at the Clinic that came my way, especially where it concerned the Prince, from the moment I ceased to be a "patient" and started working for him.* This is to show that I certainly can be trusted to be loyal and have an ironclad integrity. Unfortunately, much of the new generation is unable to comprehend that these things exist in today's social environment. The Prince forgot that I came from the Old World where trust, loyalty, and integrity were not such rare commodities.

So, to work, my gracious reader. Here comes the encounter with the medical establishment, supposedly the best. God have mercy on people who are subjected to it and triple the amount of mercy for those subject to lesser ones!

THE CASE

For three weeks now, Dr. Margaret had kept Elizabeth on muscle relaxants and stomach upset remedies. The excruciating pain in her spine and around her waist would not go away. And then on Sunday evening May 7, 1995, Elizabeth called from the bathroom:

"Come here, look at that."

I saw a discolored and slightly swollen spot about the size of a quarter above her nipple. There was a smaller spot right above it. It looked like a little boil.

"It was not here yesterday."

Cold sweat broke out on my forehead. I tried not to show any panic.

"This must be an infection, you had a clear mammogram just ten month ago, let's go to sleep and show this to Margaret in the morning."

I flew back to Rochester, to work. Elizabeth went to the doctor, and mid–day on Tuesday the doctor was on the phone.

"Mr. Sonnenberg, I am afraid I have bad news. Elizabeth's liver is in bad shape; I suspect cancer of the breast. I have sent her to the UNC Cancer Center."

Long silence.

"Hello, are you still there?"

"Yes, yes... How could we come to this state, she was under constant, supposedly first-class care?

"I do not know, apparently it happens. It must be an especially virulent type".

"Shouldn't she come off the damn hormone replacement immediately?" I said.

"Oh... yeah..,yeah..., I will tell her. Moreover, make note of the head nurse's telephone number. She will coordinate things from the Center; her name is Ms. Coolfish. Call her on Friday, they are doing tests."

I frantically started collecting all the papers, articles, and booklets Peter left around in my office. Peter who suffered from kidney cancer always brought in his latest discovery from the libraries or the special Russian bookstore in New York. I used to toss the information into a corner hoping never to have to read it myself.

On Friday, Ms. Coolfish herself called. The date was May 15, 1995.

"Mr. Sonnenberg, we finished the tests. Your wife has breast cancer and it has spread to the liver, spine, and ribs. We are admitting her to the hospital for treatment on the weekend. You must be on the plane immediately and notify your family to be here at her bed right away".

"What is the prognosis; can anything be done?" I asked.

"The prognosis is six months at the most, it is incurable, and not much we can do."

"I will fly out tonight."

I stopped by the medical center where Elizabeth was being cared for to ask Dr. De'Ignotutti for the mammogram done ten months earlier. I now saw him for the first time when he motioned me into his office with a broad swing of his arm. I saw a short, squat bulk of a man with an overhanging belly. He sat in front of me on the edge of his chair. His bloodshot eyes looked into space past my head.

"What can I do for you?"

My God, why didn't I check this guy out myself? Our family doctor had always assured me that he was recommended as being one of the best. This could not possibly be! A belly like his takes over the brain, in addition, those bloodshot eyes! The brain must be signaling red distress alert to the outside world.

"Elizabeth is in bad shape; I need the mammogram to take with me." I said.

"What is wrong?" He asked.

I told him.

"Ugh..." Was his response

That is all I could get out of him besides a rocking motion of his oversize head with its much-neglected coiffure.

We checked into the hospital on Saturday, Elizabeth in bed numb in disbelief, moving in and out of crying. I sat there trying to console her but my thoughts were far away in a desperate effort to generate a plan of action. We waited for Dr. Hope until almost midnight. I also refer to him as the **Prince**– Principal Doctor. He was a tall, lanky man in his early forties, handsome, somber-faced no smiles or friendliness for display. All my perception antennas went up – I must have turned into an info sponge. A lot was riding on the character of this man, his professional aptitude notwithstanding. As he sat down to talk to us, I observed his mannerisms as much as his words. His words came slowly, deliberately, and specifically addressed the "protocol" he chose. There was no arrogance, no self-importance, not a single opening for any idleness, encouragement, or optimism to be included. Good! I know types like him, thoughtful, flexible, and ready to listen and learn. I have worked with people like this in the past, all very, very successful. My hopes went up a notch. He might allow me to work with him, and work I intended to do!

"What do you think of him, Elizabeth?"

"I like the surgeon better; he seemed to be so friendly and caring."

"Elizabeth, my first impression is that we are lucky to have gotten *him.*"

The first test came on Monday. I took to Dr. Prince my long list of supplements and compounds for Elizabeth to take. Most of them were well known compounds except a few which a pharmacy had to prepare. I went around but nobody would touch some of the items on the list. Finally, on Margaret's suggestion I went to a Mr. Harris, the specialty pharmacist.

"Sure, can do, but I need the doctor's release. If I give this stuff to you without it, I might lose my license quick".

I called Dr. Hope, prepared for a battle. Before I even finished my explanations, he said:

"O.K., I will call the pharmacy tomorrow."

My spirits went up another notch.

"Elizabeth, I think I am right about this guy."

"Oh... he simply thinks that nothing matters anymore. I overheard him talking to the head nurse and technicians when I was waiting in the lab waiting room."

"What was that?" I asked.

"He said, 'No matter what we do, she has three months at the most."

I knew she did not make that up. She had a very sharp sense of hearing and by this time, I had glanced at some gloomy statistics.

On Tuesday, our children arrived. Having the medical compounds roughly in place, we concentrated on the diet. Jack being a food expert mapped out the list together with Maria. This was no easy task since the alternative literature is full of contradictions. We settled on areas where there was approximate agreement among all the gurus. And so, the days started rolling by, each one filled with the most dreadful emotions God has chosen for a mental torture tool set.

Once both legs of our program (the alternative medicine measures and diet) started functioning we set out to answer a few nagging questions. First, how could the trusted medical establishment have allowed such a calamity to develop? What were they saying now about nutrition, and supplementation? Is Dr. Hope going to think, and try different approaches? Will he look beyond the stiff rules of the "protocols"?

The radiology lab was the first stop.

"Doc, can you show us the films of ten months ago and the latest, and explain them."

"Sure, this is what we have today. A big mass above the nipple and other smaller masses up and closer to the chest wall."

"Doc, can we now go to the film of ten months ago? Do you see anything there?"

"No, nothing, I would have been concerned with at the time. Today, knowing the history, I would investigate that place a **little bit closer,**" he said.

He showed us a slightly, almost imperceptibly lighter area up at the chest wall. I looked in silence at those pictures for a while. Disgust and cold fury welled up in me. In my engineering years, I have looked at many X-rays of aircraft parts. If those had the fuzzy quality, I saw in these mammograms, I would never have allowed an aircraft to fly. On my way out, I saw the chief radiologist.

"Doctor, this mammogram business is bordering on criminal misrepresentation. The advertisements and assurances are certainly misleading with disastrous results in case like Elizabeth's.

"Well, yes, they are not always reliable," he said.

I did not relent in the face of answers like these, which were all I could get at the Center. I faxed one of the renowned cancer specialists. This was her reply:

"Your wife developing advanced breast cancer with normal mammograms is very common. Early detection only works in about 30% of postmenopausal women and it is not uncommon for mammography to be normal and the woman still have cancer. This just proves that we need some blood test or other technique that would really be able to find cancer in an earlier form."

At this point, I tried to purge this issue from my mind. It proved impossible. One could not avoid the persistent General Electric TV ad about their mammogram technology. "*... So that our mothers, daughters and wives can live fuller and happier lives...*" and then the greatly relieved lady hugging her husband. Fooled *my* lady! My rage came up to the same level every time!

Our next task was to find out what the Cancer Center had to say about nutrition. I did not expect too much after seeing what they served Elizabeth in the hospital. Nevertheless, I asked Ms. Coolfish.

"Ms. Coolfish, are there any dietary instructions?"

"No, she can eat whatever she wants."

On my way out, I picked up one of their nutritional guide booklets. One of the first pages featured a sloppy Joe on a bun. When we went for a second opinion to a famous and competing Cancer Center, the conversation with their oncologist went as follows.

"Doctor, are there any nutritional changes we need to be making?"

"No, not at all, I can see that she is not malnourished".

"What about vitamin supplementation?"

"No, vitamins can actually be harmful."

"Which ones can be harmful?"

"Oh... vitamin A for example, could be quite toxic."

We left that center glad that we had not ended up in this overcrowded "mass production" facility, its fame notwithstanding.

We hit the books and libraries with a fury. After two weeks, armed with my naive post-graduate knowledge, I was ready to talk to the doctor. Two things were abundantly clear. Nutrition has a profound and well-documented impact, if not for a cure then certainly on the conduct of the disease. Secondly, the world of alternative approaches is overwhelmingly large and confusing. "A minefield" was the proper characterization by one of the writers.

After a few weeks passed in the intensive application of nutritional principles and supplementation, Elizabeth started to give me a hard time about it. Where could I get help? There was a counseling person at the clinic, the ever ebullient and friendly Ms. Mercy, a young, attractive woman in her late twenties, maybe a little older. She was a beaming smile, compassion, so concerned, and friendly, it seemed that crying on her shoulder was irresistible. She suggested a support group many times.

Mercy: "We have a support group here, Elizabeth should join," Mercy said.

"I will ask, but my guess is, she will not go to these crying sessions."

"Oh! They do not cry, they laugh about it."

"Well, that is sick in itself."

As I talked to Mercy, I thought maybe she can help with Elizabeth's grumbling.

"Mercy, will you talk to Elizabeth about keeping the diet?"

"Sure, I will make an appointment."

After the meeting, I asked Elizabeth, "How did it go?"

"Oh... I don't think I will talk to her again."

"Why?"

"She was asking about my plans and telling me to concentrate on nice things to do in the very little time I have left."

The rest came out the next day when Elizabeth became angry about some trifle and burst into:

"I am sick and tired of you, checking every little bite I take. I should listen to Mercy when she tells me to get you off my back and not let you run my life!"

Damn! I had better keep her away from that counselor from hell. The next scheduled meeting with Mercy fell through and from that time on she faded out of our sight, but not from my mind. I decided to concentrate on my studies and my relationship with the doctor.

Three weeks passed and it was time to see him.

"Elizabeth, we will schedule some more chemos now".

"You scheduled only one initially, doctor?"

"Yes, I did not expect you to survive the first."

After the second chemo he called me one evening:

"Sven, have you seen Elizabeth's blood test?"

"Yes Doc, I wish the GGT (one of the crucial liver enzymes) was better."

"Man, don't you know that this GGT is as if she'd 2 drinks too many the previous night?"

Yes, I knew, but nothing was good enough for me. I must have expected a miracle.

"I can tell you now that patients in Elizabeth's condition, as it has been, we have lost very fast."

As time progressed, my positive feelings for the doctor became ever stronger. Occasionally, I would take what I thought were applicable papers to him. He would respond after reading, always attentive, relevant and always at my level, never from above. He even made time for me on Saturday after his hospital rounds. After seeing one paper, which concerned a crucial issue in chemotherapy, he said, "Hardly a conference or seminar passes without us discussing this subject."

"This means that we will soon come to the chemo's limitation and then there is no chance for chasing that cancer out."

"Some revelation," he must have thought. However, he said, "Well, after the chemo there is tamoxifen which can keep the cancer in check."

"Doc, can you experiment? Suppose you decide to abandon the protocol and go your own way. Can you do it?" *(Please refer to page 60 or below "Best doctors in America)*

"Yes, but I would have to justify that and get the agreement of the national coordinator."

"Where is that coordinator?"

"Bethesda"

That confirmed my fears, that we would be stuck in "protocols" none of which offered any hope, real hope, for long–term improvement.

Elizabeth, though, got progressively better. The trips to the Center for chemo application, depressing in themselves, made us aware of how different Elizabeth's condition was. The chemo subjects were suffering hell –

diarrhea, vomiting, and infections. Some ended up in the hospital with severe infections after every chemo. Elizabeth was sailing through with mild discomfort. The doctor's only twitch of curiosity as to "why" would be his comment:

"Elizabeth is doing incredibly well under the chemo!"

Whenever I made more adjustments to the horrendous amount of pills she was taking, I showed them to the doctor. I was always afraid that he would object and ask me to desist or reduce. This time, I flashed the list before him, trying to have it both ways, for him to see but not to see too well.

"Hey, let me look at this, I need to see the dosages!" he said when I tried to take the list back.

He looked at it line-by-line, top to bottom and said nothing at first. I did not know whether to be glad or concerned. I was dreaming that he would "employ" me to do some research work on novel material or relevant papers. I would not be a nuisance! When he mentioned a new drug in the pipeline and heading toward clinical trials already for 3 years now, I asked him again to give me some work to find out more and hit the trail after it, to no avail. The doctor's only reaction to my list was:

"With such high doses of C you will give the lady kidney stones."

"Doc, this is the least of my worries, under the circumstances."

"Yeah...Yeah."

He looked some more.

"You might up the selenium a little bit."

Yes, Sir..ehhh ... Doctor."

"Maybe I should put you in touch with Ms. Gourmet, she is on our staff and tries to bring us around to this stuff, and she is very persistent."

"Oh... Doc, this would be fantastic. Can I have her name and telephone number?"

"I will make the arrangements."

He never did, although I reminded him twice. He even put it down on his yellow memo pad. His failure to do this could not have been forgetfulness or a coincidence. This was the beginning of the end of my naive enchantment with the Clinic's operation. Being awed by all that complexity in the operation of the Clinic, I was extremely concerned not to offend his or anybody else's sensitivity, in an attempt to not even subconsciously weaken the doctor's attention to Elizabeth's case. Therefore, I was in a quandary every time my thrashing around took me to some area outside the "Protocol", hoping to find some other treatment than that horrendous chemo. One day, again in an acute state of anxiety, I took up the invitation from the caring and friendly surgeon Elizabeth liked so much to talk, though I wondered if Dr. Hope would be offended by my talking with his colleague. The surgeon had just recently received his doctorate in immunity.

"Doc, there is such confusion about immunity and cancer. Some say it fights the disease, others say it does not. What is your opinion?"

"Both parties are wrong, some cancers are fought by the immune system, others are not. The breast is one where the immune system is impotent."

"But Doc, how is it that the cancer, having such proliferatory power and rapid growth, is often kept in check without intervention for a considerable time?

"If I knew the answer to this I would be on the plane to Sweden to pick up the Nobel `Prize."

As I prodded and kept up my search, of which Dr. Hope was generally aware, our meetings became less frequent and shorter. It came to the point where I had to beg repeatedly for a meeting, only to be told by the secretary, "OK, Friday morning, 15 minutes, no more."

Elizabeth improved in the meantime to the point where some residual cancer was still visible but the chemo was reaching "a plateau", a euphemism for it being no longer effective. I was expecting to hear soon, "Time to gracefully exit the "protocol" and go on to tamoxifen." By this time, I became obsessed with my relationship with Dr. Hope. I could not stop speculating in my mind about what environment he was working in. He was obviously different from the other doctors. We confirmed that by talking to the patients of other doctors. There were also many little clues. One time we stayed late at the Clinic, mostly waiting. The place was empty, except for Dr. Hope's assistant, Teresa, and ourselves.

"Teresa, it is past seven and you are still here?"

"Yeah... if you are with Dr. Hope that is what you have to endure."

Or:

"Nurse, is this test included?"

"Yeah, yeah, with Dr. Hope you always get that!"

A few days later, we learned that in the competing center where we had gone for second opinion oncologists see from 40 to 50 patients a day. I wondered if our Dr. Hope was an outcast for not fulfilling his *quota*? Is he under some pressure from the bureaucracy or his peers? Are my activities adding to his difficulties? Other patients, as we learned, do whatever the doctor says; they stay on the beaten path, which is littered with corpses, until they too end up a statistic. Some silently drop out and go milling around in a mostly futile search for someone to help them. Since it seemed that any further "imposition" on my part was only leading to a "soft" indifference, I decided to see him and made a speech as follows:

Dear Dr. Hope,

I have this to say today.

I will begin by saying that we are very grateful to you for all you have done for Elizabeth. Without your special attention, effort and flexibility her improvement would not have been possible. However, the published statistics and my own - a poor man's statistics- are not good. I can only believe that Elizabeth's remission is pretty exceptional. Following the success achieved so far, I aspire to try to totally chase the cancer out. I know that this is considered impossible by the established canons of today's medicine. Therefore, I have the difficult dilemma facing me now as to whether to try to prepare some contingent actions or rest on the current improvement. It is my nature not to take the passive route. I feel that nothing should be changed as long as there is continuing improvement, but I probably will be searching the universe of clinical trials and alternative methods. Very often, there are trials, which are local and not known to other cancer centers or even the NCI. Recently I came across one of those.

My main purpose in my visit today is to ask for reassurances that you will continue to give us your full support. So far, I have not found anything worth bringing to your attention. Should I find something and the situation calls for unusual action, I would like to count on your help to get into a trial, or if it is not something on the beaten track I would plead with you to stay with us and give your evaluation and support. It is possible that by doing so other patients may benefit besides Elizabeth.

I am absolutely convinced that there are constraints flowing from your medical environment –peer interactions, rules from the NCI, coordinators and what have you. It is not possible for me to guess what they might be. I would plead with you again to be frank and open so that I do not charge off in a direction that will cause trouble or aggravate the situation.

My speech was received in a polite manner and my understanding was that he would continue to support us unconditionally. His comments concerning the speech were as follows:

"I agree with your statement that Elizabeth's case is exceptional, but I strongly disagree with you, that the statistics are dismal. There are some 5% to 10% of cases where people live a considerable time."

I did not ask what, in his opinion would be dismal.

Next, he sketched some possibilities in relating to my "aspirations", or so I guessed. These were all very toxic mainstream "protocols", including the "dandy" bone marrow transplantation. This is used after wiping the patient out by harsh chemo and then resuscitating him by rebuilding the destroyed bone marrow. There was only one non-toxic alternative, for which, it turned out later, Elizabeth was not eligible. I did not ask if he recommended these harsher measures now!

I thought this is the end of my efforts to shake him loose from the mainstream bureaucratic "protocols". Nevertheless, my speculations about his inner thinking continued unabated. Does he believe that the methods used by the clinic are the only correct approaches? This cannot be! Number one, he is too open–minded and too smart. All that these methods do is prolong life a bit, often a life of very poor quality. Does he think that these treatments are the best available, everything else is thin ice? Does he consciously go along with the flow - no controversial moves – because this secures a career path? I can understand a decision like that.

To experiment with Elizabeth or any other patient on his own would mean groans, squeaks, and continuous controversy from the "well-oiled" machinery of the clinic. Moreover, what about the High Priest Coordinator! One should not forget the fear of lawsuits, once outside official bounds. I may be expecting too much! Such a course could mean disaster to one's career. In my working years, I was cautiously rebellious but not enough for greatness, and I know the agony, of not having the reckless compulsion to follow one's own trail. I said to him in writing, trying to induce him into something extraordinary:

"...We have already observed qualities in you that make a superb foundation for outstanding achievements..."

What chutzpah from a lowly patient! He told me he was not offended!

I came across a relevant passage in an outstanding book; The Savage Cell by Pat McGrady. These words were written 32 years ago, in 1964:

> *... Occasionally a Scientist bucks the system and does notable work. He is taken care of. They make him head of a department [if he is not fired or ostracized– S.S.], dean, chancellor, president of the university, in which position he is burdened with administrative duties, money raising, handshaking, and speechmaking so that he never again enters a laboratory,*

I had better count the blessings we have received from Dr. Hope and go. I must keep us in his good graces though, if it comes, destiny forbid, to a bone marrow transplant!

I redoubled my efforts to find some reasonable alternative. I read, wrote, faxed, and tried to reach authors of cancer–related papers. A typical conversation would go as follows:

"Professor, I read your article in such and such publication is there any practical activity going on in your institution related to the method you describe?"

"Not that I know of, this is all in the early research phase. Besides, I am not a clinician so I could not help you anyway. Talk to so and so."

These activities and sending for and interpreting obscure tests, which no cancer center heard of, took most of my days.

By this time it was fall 1996, more than a year had passed from the time of Elizabeth's predicted death. All that time she was without any physical impairment or even the slightest pain, and for all practical purposes leading a "normal" life. After tamoxifen was started, some side effects showed up, but nothing debilitating. Elizabeth took this as an excuse for skipping items from our routine list. In addition, forbidden foods started showing up on the table. Her mood swings became worse. Not a whole lot worse though than in the past, before her illness. Her anger was always very close to the surface. Any displeasure or seeming provocation brought out a nasty outburst. Once I said, "Elizabeth, all these years I have never heard an apology for the nasty things you sometimes come up with."

"I am too perfect to apologize for anything."

"Granted, nearly perfect you are, but in the department of bridling your anger you are sometimes lacking."

"You have an uncommon wife. Besides a husband is also for venting one's frustrations."

Just recently, I saw a Frank Sinatra film. Sinatra visits his heart–attack-stricken father. In the ensuing emotional conversation, Frank, frustrated with his relations with women, asks his dad, "Dad, how come you and Mom lasted all these years?"

"Son, I do not listen and I do not speak."

Had I adopted that philosophy, our thirty-six years together would have been smoother.

One day one of the more recent tests came, a test not ordered by the clinic but ordered through our holistic doctor. (These activities of mine were not paid for by our insurance.)

"I think all that activity of yours is nothing but making work for you. You are spending money and I suffer all this jerking around. Next time you intend to make an appointment or a test, I want to approve it beforehand. Moreover, every other day I see some new pills. I've had enough of this!" Elizabeth said.

Now, this was a blow at precisely the wrong distance, below the belt. All the agony of fear and pain I had been in, and was going through! I guessed I would not see the full effect of my "adjuvant therapy."

"Elizabeth, have your own way from now on."

A CT scan and a doctor's review visit were coming up. As usual, I was preparing and agonizing about this and that. This time, I was debating whether to give the doctor the whole program list, diet, references, and schedules, all neatly printed out. He knew most of it but not in the form of such a detailed document. After the latest outburst from Elizabeth, the much of the wind had gone out of my sails, but I decided to go through the motions nevertheless.

The tests and scans showed the same lesions in the liver as before.

"Radiology has concluded that there is no change. To me it looks like a slight improvement. You know, it may be scar lesions but we have to assume it is still cancer," Dr. Hope said.

Then he started filling out the usual papers and schedules for future checks. In the middle of this, he said, as if to himself:

"This is certainly an ATYPICAL case!"

Did I detect a slight note of disappointment, or satisfaction? I did not know which. Of course, I knew what his words meant, but I asked anyway.

"What do you mean by that, Doc?"

"Well, by this time the cancer is usually back in full force and we start the merry- go-round with chemos again."

At the end of the visit, I handed him the folder.

"Doc, I have a feeling, not supported by any logic, that this should be for your eyes only, but you must be the judge of what to do with it."

He looked it over and said, "How many pills is she taking a day now?"

"Eighty–five or so."

"Make sure she drinks a lot throughout the day."

"Yes, Doc."

31

He took the folder and held it up in his right hand, as if hesitating over what to do with it.

"I will put it into Elizabeth's file right at the end, with the other stuff you gave me. We will refer to it as the **Contra Program.**"

"I guess, Doc, that nobody looks at that file but you, anyway."

"That is right. Any other questions?"

"Yes."

Before I started with the question, he said:

"I have spent some time on that Zeneca [*supposedly a better drug than tamoxifen –S.S.*], and I think some commercialism is going on here, I hear different stories from different people in that outfit. It does not look as if they will release it soon since they have just released this other thing." [*Much inferior, they spent a lot of developing money I would guess–S.S*]

"Doc, let me go after them."

"Give me one month without interference and then we will talk."

"Yes, Doc."

In December, Dr. Hope concluded that the chemotherapy had reached a "plateau." No more improvement could be seen on the MRIs (Magnetic Resonance Imaging).

"It is time to gracefully exit CAF (one of the combination chemotherapy protocols) and go on Tamoxifen."

Elizabeth went on Tamoxifen in January, 1996. The months following were full of side effects never heard of by Dr. Hope. Shoulder pains, fatigue. These did not go away after the expected duration of a few weeks. I was reading and bringing to Dr. Hope all the bad reports about Tamoxifen from Lancet and elsewhere. He would only say:

"There is a shrill movement in some quarters against Tamoxifen, all these reports are vastly exaggerated. There is another drug in the pipeline that is supposed to not have some of these side effects. I keep mentioning this to you and to some of my other patients unresponsive to Tamoxifen. This has been going on for three years now and the drug has not been brought out yet. The company is Zeneca and the drug has a preliminary designation of Zeneca182780."

I was uneasy and worried. Granted, Tamoxifen is now in wide use and as usual, there is only a certain small percentage of disastrous side effect cases.

Nevertheless, if one is lucky... Tamoxifen, at its best, promised only one to three years of effectiveness. After that, the cancer becomes resistant. From "my" statistics, the response time lasted three to twenty months. I now started investigating the Zeneca situation. The drug was far from FDA approval, but one hospital in Manchester, UK, conducted a trial with "encouraging" results. What "encouraging" means in their parlance is that out of 19 patients 13 "responded" after Tamoxifen failure. That further breaks down to seven having partial responses and six showing no change. That lasted 18 months. What was more important, no adverse effect on the liver was found, unlike Tamoxifen, which affects the liver, sometimes disastrously. I tried to induce Dr. Hope to get this drug for Elizabeth and his other patients on a humanitarian basis. All my cajoling and proposals for action with me assembling a group of needy patients to petition the authorities ended in Dr. Hope finding out what the official plans for the drug were. Double blind randomized trials against Tamoxifen. Since Elizabeth already was on Tamoxifen she was obviously not eligible. This was one of many meetings with Dr. Hope:

"Doc, can I contact the other patients who need Zeneca?"

"I cannot give out that information. This is a privacy matter, and if I did, I could be fired. What I can do is contact them individually and ask for permission and then you can go!"

"That is fantastic, when can you do it?"

"I think with Rebecca's help making the list I can have it by Saturday."

That Saturday never came.

Sure enough, Elizabeth's liver enzymes started to go up in September 1996, which was nine months of the so-called NC (no change). Since Tamoxifen alone can cause the enzymes to go up substantially, I was hoping for that to be the case. The CT scan told us otherwise. The cancer in the liver had started "progressing." The other sites, the bones, and breasts were clear, with no new sites elsewhere.

"Tamoxifen isn't working. What is left now is Taxol. I am sorry. We really do not have anything better."

He handed Elizabeth a consent form.

"Doctor, is there hair loss involved again?" Elizabeth asked.

"Oh... yes."

"Then I do not want it, I would agree if this was a cure but to go through all that again, and end up at the same point, no."

"Doc, what about Megaze? Could we try it for a short while and see? Would that be reasonable?" I asked.

"Yes, we can do that. If it does not work, we could perhaps try Navelbine, which is a milder chemo. She may not lose her hair."

Elizabeth went on Megaze in October, 1996.

I also pursued another track. From the very beginning, I tried to find a non– toxic approach, preferably an immunological one. After much phoning, I found Dr. Alternate in San Diego that very October. However, those people would not talk to an engineer; they demanded that Dr. Hope call.

"Doc, I found this trial in San Diego, but they will not talk to me. Will you please call Dr. Alternate and see if there is anything worthwhile there?"

"O.K. Give me the material. I will study it and give you an answer at the next visit."
At the next meeting, he said, "I think they may have something there. I will talk to Dr. Alternate."

In January 1997, after three month of Megaze, the CT scan showed further "progression" in the liver. Dr. Hope had not yet spoken to Dr. Alternate and I became desperate. I called Manchester and reached one of the Zeneca trial doctors. Dr. Howell agreed to talk to me from his sick–bed at home.

"Doc, in your opinion, is that drug worth me going all the way out to England for, should I chain myself to the company gate in Manchester?

"No, this Faslodex [*by this time it had a brand name-S.S.*] is uncharted territory. On the other hand, you should not allow her liver to decompose and it will, if you wait too long. Under the circumstances, I suggest Taxotere. It has a 50% response rate. Nevertheless, I can give you the name of the principal investigator at Zeneca. You can call him and ask for compassionate release, but I doubt if they will go along."

"Thank you, Doctor."

"Are you a practicing oncologist?"

"No, Doctor, I am an engineer."

"Please do not be offended by my question, it is fine with me. I was just curious."

That was a nice surprise coming from an Englishman. I had to revise my stereotyping of the English as being a haughty, arrogant bunch because of this courteous and professional treatment I received from England four times in a row. They never failed to call me back promptly when I left a message.

"I understand that doctors in the USA have a little more time for their patients".

"Well, Doctor, our oncologist has upwards of 600 patients, and hardly any time."

"I wish I had 600 hundred; I have double that."

The conversation ended with me thanking him profusely in genuine gratitude. I now turned away from Zeneca and called San Diego, asking Elizabeth to be admitted to their immunological clinical trial. They finally accepted information from me, but all the formal work and preparation had to be done by Dr. Hope, and in the meantime, Elizabeth went without any treatment. Dr. Hope's secretary was useless.

"Teresa, if Dr. Hope does not call Dr. Alternate today, I am coming over with a sleeping bag and I will camp in front of his office."

That started things rolling, but only a bit. At our next visit, I said, "I have talked to San Diego. We will make the necessary preparations. Doc, did you talk to Dr. Alternate?"

"No, I talked to his coordinating nurse, Denise."

"Did you get the proper information; is it worthwhile to try it? We need your opinion and judgment."

"Yes, it is legitimate and worthwhile, and this is the time to try it."

On February 4, 1997, we showed up at Dr. Alternate's office across the full width of the continental USA with a full load of documentation and a letter of recommendation from Dr. Hope.

Dr. Alternate looked at the CT scans and the rest of the documents and said:

"The immunological program is not suitable for Elizabeth's condition. The liver situation is too advanced for my program to be effective. Anyway, we are just at the beginning of this approach, and so far, we have had some no- change responses in very small lesions. In other cases we have had no responses."
After a short pause, he continued:

"In Elizabeth's condition, where the liver is the problem and the other sites are in remission and quiescent, it does not make sense to expose the whole system to these horrible toxins. I propose liver chemoembolization (treating the liver locally with a combination of chemo drugs). We are doing this procedure a lot at our clinic with a fair amount of success. If you want to do it here, fine, if not, I am sure other places can do it too."

"Do you think that our clinic in Carolina has that capability?"

"If not in Chapel Hill then perhaps someplace close".

I called Dr. Hope.

"Doc, this immunological approach isn't what it seemed to be, they are proposing chemoembolization."

"Oh... we have that here too. If you come back, we will do an evaluation under Dr. Cunningnerd. If Elizabeth qualifies, then it can be done in about two weeks."

"But, Doc, we can hardly wait; we need to decide now what to do!"

"Sven, I have to run, call me on Friday, late, we can discuss this in detail then."

I turned to Dr. Alternate.

"Doc, we cannot mess around any longer. Please do it, if Elizabeth agrees. Will you please talk to Dr. Hope and explain the situation. I am afraid he may get offended, we need his continuing support."

"Very well, I agree, we should not delay, I will arrange things for Monday and I will also talk to Dr. Hope. They ought to give you full cooperation back in Chapel Hill. If not, you should find somebody else."

Find somebody else! That is like saying: Go find a needle in a rotting haystack.

Therefore, Elizabeth underwent the procedure in San Diego on February 10, 1997. Her recovery from the aftermath of that procedure was long and frightening. The weakness and low hemoglobin caused Dr. Hope to be concerned about her iron deficiency. Sure enough, it turned out that she was deficient. The iron sulfate pills taken over the weekend for that made her suffering worse. Alarmed, I used every means to get the doctor to return my call, to no avail for the entire week. Next Tuesday we had a visit.

"Doctor, I had a scare on Monday, could not reach you through your secretary or assistant. Your beeper did not work either. Things are deteriorating at the clinic. I have given her some molasses. I am very concerned about the iron; she should not take any more than necessary to restore the physiological level. Excess iron is bad for cancer. I have it from reliable sources."

"Well, I have given you more time than other patients get. If you do not like it here, I suggest you go somewhere else. In addition, that iron test, I have not ordered it this time and I am not interested in it. You should pay for it out of your own pocket."

"Doc, I was hoping that you would never say such things."

After that, the visit ended with a routine "see you in two weeks" and a promise that at that time the iron would be checked. Molasses was approved - "If she can tolerate it." At the next visit, there was no mention of the iron test. We still did not know whether that iron load continued to be necessary and I did not raise the issue. We would go to our holistic doctor and ask him to do a lab test.

There were two more embolizations, April 14 and June 16 of the same year. After the April treatment, recovery went well. Spirits were high because of that, and the effectiveness of the earlier treatment was good. The third, June 16, that was supposedly a "touch up" ended badly. Three days after checking out of San Diego's Perlman Center Elizabeth's bowels shut down completely. We learned later that this is a common effect of morphine and codeine. The latter is used liberally as a painkiller. On April 23, Elizabeth went into uncontrollable shivering, and on arriving in the ER at UCLA Medical Center her blood pressure measured 50/38. This time I was impressed by the staff's approach. Nothing was left unchecked. This was also the first time pleural (lung cavity) fluid was detected and drained. I took the opportunity to find out if UCLA had something to offer for the cancer. All I heard was "Taxol, no more embolizations, we can apply the first treatment here, if you wish."

"No thank you Dr. Rosove. We will wait until our return to Carolina."

Dr. Rosove was a "swift fellow" of an oncologist, shooting back answers before I could finish my questions. He was so expert and sure of himself! I asked Elizabeth, "Would you like to be in his care?"

"No way!"

That took care of UCLA. Most of the other people involved in Elizabeth's case made an outstanding impression. I usually started my contact with this:

"I know you do not like engineers, but..."

"Oh... no, that is not the case!"

From that point on things usually went agreeably, and people were forthcoming.

Toward the end of August 1997, tests showed that the breast and the bones were flaring up again. Elizabeth developed shortness of breath and became bloated. The findings were: in addition to the pleural effusion, there was a bad case of ascites. From that point on events started rolling fast. Initially, the tests showed no malignant cells on site, on the lung or abdomen. I was told, "That does not mean that there are no cancer implants. Malignant cells are detected only in about 75% of cases, although cancer exists."

Elizabeth was drained repeatedly and toward the end of September 97 underwent the sclerosis procedure (attaching the lung to the rib cage so that the accumulation of fluid is prevented). She was back in the Hospital; the Prince was away and the attending physician was Dr. Cunningnerd. I remembered that the Prince had mentioned that he would drain the fluid before applying systemic chemo, and the choice was of course Taxol. I went to Cunningnerd.

"Doc, Elizabeth is bloated, and has a lot of fluid in the abdomen. I was told that maybe it should be drained before the Taxol. The chemo may sit there and not be eliminated."

"No, we will take care of that later; the fluid does not prevent us from going ahead. It is not remaining in the fluid."

She received Taxol on September 30, 1997. I watched her neutrophils drop every day until they reached 0.5. I started going from doctor to doctor on the floor asking that they give her G-CSF (this is a white cell growth stimulant). To no avail. On the fourth day, the situation had become desperate. Her neutrophil count dropped to ZERO and she developed paralytic ileus. The parade of doctors feeling and listening to Elizabeth's abdomen was increasing by the hour.

"It is gas. The bowels are not working, and we cannot use an enema because of fear of infection since her white cell count is low."

The torture Elizabeth went through with the nose catheter, and IVs, etc. was excruciating. On the fourth day, she got the G-CSF stimulation. It was too late. A blood infection had set in and now the antibiotics were rolled out. To top it, the Prince on his return from his trip concluded that it was not gas, but fluid and she needed to be drained. Elizabeth came out of this a ruin.

Her inner ear balance nerves had been damaged by the combination of Taxol and the antibiotic Gentamicin, and she was emaciated, a skeleton. As might be expected, nobody, the Prince included, knew how to handle the loss of balance. An outside neurological specialist, after charging an exorbitant fee for a 15 minutes consultation said, "This is a toughie." Therefore, we were left to our own" devices." The brain CT scan did not show any reason for the condition. The Prince's comment:

"That is not good news. By now I would not be surprised if it had spread to the brain."

I realized that Cunningnerd had screwed up badly. It was not even an honest mistake, but incompetence and neglect. I debated, "what should one do in such a situation?" Run to a lawyer? Complain? Go elsewhere? None of these options seemed feasible certainly not a protracted lawsuit with Elizabeth in her condition, a lawsuit that probably could not be won because the doctors would hide behind "protocols." What could we accomplish? Would we harm or help Elizabeth? Perhaps it would only worsen the existing situation and drain our desperately needed resources. I resolved to watch and check every little move they made from then on.

It was very difficult to react on the spot to every little instruction from them. I had to study and do research to evaluate what their utterances meant. In an instance where even a short waiting time is permissible, this would be O.K. What should I do in fast-moving situations where I have to rely totally on their judgment? I can imagine how inscrutable their incorrect treatments are with the average patient. What a perfect situation they have in which to do just anything without anybody recognizing their misdeeds or punishing them except in the most dramatically obvious cases! We said to the Prince. "From now on we ask that any decision of importance be made only with your explicit oversight and approval." Without asking any questions, with his head down, not even looking up from his papers, he said, "O.K."

Elizabeth started a slow recuperation process from the Taxol disaster. Toward the end of November, the Prince started talking about Navelbine. A much gentler chemo, should be no problem.

"We will see to it, that you are able to go Los Angeles for the holidays to see your son".

With great hope we started Navelbine on December 2, 1997. The consequences were immediate and disastrous. Paralysis of the intestinal tract, complete blockage and vomiting of blood. She was in and out of the emergency room with abdominal pain from the ascities and constipation, low blood pressure after parenthesis (abdominal draining); fevers et cetera, et cetera. Again the prescription laxatives and anti-nausea prescription drugs made the situation worse. Her liver enzymes went out of sight. We stopped all this after a few days and went to our holistic doctor. Slowly, by using those maligned remedies from the health food store with primary reliance on Aloe Vera juice, Elizabeth's intestines started to function again. But by that time she was a skeleton barely able to move because of weakness and the loss of balance.

The Prince said he had to think it over and he would propose something. Toward the end of December, he started talking 5-FU, the only thing left in the "arsenal," considering Elizabeth's reaction to previous measures and the presence of ascites that prevented the use of some of the other chemos,. The decision then came down that it was going to be 5-FU on January 8, 1998. On January 8 he changed his mind, saying that we had to take care of the ascites somehow. He proposed a Denver shunt (a tube from the abdomen back into the blood circulatory system). He set up a meeting with a surgeon, Dr. Malvor, to discuss that. This is part of the conversation with Dr. Malvor.

"Doc, how many of these operation do you do?"

"Not many. In fact I perform them very rarely."

"But you must have a lot of patients with ascites?"

"Yes, but they die fast, and it is not right to put them through the trauma of surgery for a benefit of very short duration. Elizabeth's situation is unusual, and that is why we are talking."

The Prince told us much the same during our January 8 visit. At that time he said he would be absent from the clinic for three weeks so we would talk on January 27. That meant that nothing would happen, and Elizabeth would be without any treatment or attention for that time. From that visit on, I sensed a change in the Prince's attitude. Once again, he mentioned that he was giving us more time than he gave other patients. He did not call us at home one single time during the three weeks. Previously he had checked on Elizabeth's status sporadically. Each time I was elated, because it is uncommon these days for any Doctor to show even a shred of humanity. It also made me think that he was interested in our case for the sake of medical science and that gave me so much comfort. Now the visits became short, with not much deliberation or inquiry about what we were doing ourselves concerning alternatives. His interest was obviously waning. This tells me volumes about that "profession." An engineer would act in exactly the opposite way, with a case to learn from, his interest would be piqued, and the tests and exploration of "why" would intensify. Not with these guys though.

In that three-week "interlude" I started calling doctors from the Best Doctor organization list. I also called Dr. Alternate in San Diego. The contact from Dr. Alternate's office in San Antonio told me to send the abdominal fluid for cell culturing to see which standard or investigational drug would work. I arranged that without the Prince's participation. The contact in Miami, Dr. Vogel, thought it a good idea to test Elizabeth for blood HER2/neu. If she was positive, the monoclonal antibody treatment could be tried. I had asked the Prince to test her for that more than a year ago and it had come in negative. That is why I disregarded all trials using that approach. January 27 came.

"Hi Sven, I have talked to your Internet buddy, Dr. Vogel. I think we should test Elizabeth again for HER2/neu. This treatment is quite effective."

"When?"

"I have to find out how to go about it, give me two days."

"Doctor, I have also sent the fluid to San Antonio, to Dr. Van Hoff."

"Oh... Yes, I know Dr. Van Hoff. Good man! This will help me determine if we need to change the course of treatment."

Nothing much more happened on January 27, except a promise to talk to Dr. Candrill about checking Elizabeth's portal vein pressure to see if the ascites had a contributing factor from portal vein hypertension. This was a follow–up of my initiative when I went to Dr. Candrill and asked him to investigate. The portal vein pressure test was done on February 3. Sure enough, there was a degree of elevated pressure. That same day I asked the Prince, "When will Elizabeth have that HER2/neu test?"

"Why don't you find out where it is done from Dr. Vogel."

Two days later, I had the information. I went to the Prince on Thursday to ask, what next?

"We will draw the blood tomorrow, send it to Dianon. I am also on my way to Dr. Candrill to discuss the liver test results and his findings. We will decide what to do, if anything. Then we should start the 5-FU. I will let you know in 48 hours."

The blood was drawn. Our lab could not handle it because the FDA had not approved the test yet. Dianon in New Jersey would not accept the order without a valid account from the hospital. Next, I found out that the Prince had an account at Dianon.

At this point a number of questions were swirling in my head. First, the Prince had known about San Antonio and Dr. Van Hoff but had never said a word. The test in San Antonio seemed to be of crucial importance to the case, certainly after the "standard" chemos failed or the cells became resistant to them. In any case it seems unconscionable not to explore what, and if any, agent has an impact on cancer cells as soon as feasible instead of blindly relying on protocols. Secondly, what about the HER2/neu test? Where and how was it done before? Was it done at all? Had it been done properly, but later the cells had mutated? Should there not be a periodic test to see if HER2/cell expression increases during the course of the illness? An engineer in my employ would be severely censored for missing issues similar to these.

The 48 hours passed without a word. A long Monday, no word. On Tuesday I called Dianon. They were not allowed to give results to me. Now it was Thursday, still no word. I started speculating. Has the Prince given up on Elizabeth? Is he angry with me and taking it out on her? Do these guys, when they see their patient in what they perceive is a hopeless condition want to finish him or her quickly by silent withdrawal of treatment? Have they a pact with the insurance companies and are they practicing passive euthanasia? What is the matter with him? I ran to the clinic to ask for the HER2/NEU results and to tell him: Elizabeth cannot wait any longer without treatment. He saw me and with absolute casualness said, "The HER2/NEU is elevated. She might be eligible for the lottery to enter treatment, why don't you contact Dr. Vogel? As far as the 5 - FU, I will arrange it right away. Come tomorrow for the port implantation."

He was most unperturbed, not mentioning what had transpired with Dr. Candrill or what had been said a week ago. He did not comment about or express interest in the fact that the cancer cells from Elizabeth's abdominal fluid were not growing in the culture at Dr. Van Hoff's lab in San Antonio. The 5-FU treatment turned out to be on February 16, and the next appointment with the Prince was on February 17. Elizabeth would then have been more than two and half-months without treatment.

Julia arrived with the 5-FU pump and the rest of the equipment.

"Julia, what is the prescribed dose?"

"$300mg/m^2$, which works out to $460mg/24$ hours for Elizabeth."

"Is this a high dose or what?"

"No, it is medium; sometimes we apply $600mg/m^2$. So, it is just in the middle."

I took this at face value, trusting that the Prince knew what he was doing. Woe is me! The only thing I did was to look up what she had been given in the CAF combination. It was a $200mg/m^2$ one-time infusion. So, I thought, maybe that 300 is okay over a 24-hour period.

After three days of a 460mg of 5-FU a day she was in a horrible condition. Her mouth became one big sore. She stopped eating. Whenever I tried to force any food on her, she would go into uncontrollable sobbing. The growing ascites and associated problems made the situation unbearable. During that week, from Monday to the next Monday the Prince did not call once to inquire if the dose was too high! That Monday Elizabeth had a severe case of mucositis (severe inflammation of the mouth and throat lining). She was vomiting blood, could not swallow, and could not speak. In short, she was headed for the hospital. For three days in the hospital she did not eat one morsel. I became concerned and expressed that concern loudly. Eventually they installed a TPN (Total Parenteral Nutrition) bag.

"What is in that mixture?"

"Oh…. Vitamins, amino acids, and fat. A good nutritional mix."

My goodness! Was this a mixture?! Her liver enzymes went through the roof. When the nurses drew blood, they marveled at the streaks of fat floating in the tube.

"We have seen this only with very obese people or ones that have gorged on some fatty foods, like a lot of quarter pounder hamburgers before the blood draw".

On the fifth day, Elizabeth was doing a little better, after pain and anti-nausea medication were stopped on my insistence. Quite obviously, these worked at cross-purposes. The pain medication induced vomiting and the anti- nausea treatment caused stomach irritation and pain. They applied Fluconasole with my great misgivings, but I agreed, thinking that maybe, one application would not harm her and in the meantime I would study it. We would stop it if I found something wrong. That Fluconasole must have hit her liver hard, for she ended up in the intensive care unit one hour after that ill–begotten infusion. The next day her liver enzymes started to really go out of sight. Dr. Broth, the liver specialist, appeared.

"Ah... Dr. Broth, are you the liver specialist?"

"Yes"

"How much time do you have to talk?"

"Five minutes."

"Five minutes?!"

"I have spent half an hour reviewing her paperwork!"

"Then you have seen the liver enzyme report!

"Yes"

"The ALT and AST have gone down in range since February 16. GGT is half and ALP is half. Did you see that? What do you think happened? I would expect them to go temporarily higher after the chemo."

I did not tell him that Elizabeth had been on alpha lipoic acid just before the start of the chemo, this was on Dr. Fine's suggestion — our alternative guy, because I could see that all the enzymes were drifting higher every new blood test.

"Well, the enzyme situation is a very complex one. The ALT and AST may have gone down because there are no functional liver cells left."

"Doc, did you also see that after yesterday's application of Fluconasole the same enzymes shot up to highs never seen before?"

"That is the result of the TPN. There is a lot of fat in that formula and it puts a burden on the liver."

Why the non-existent liver cells produced that much variation in enzyme levels was not explained. This kind of logic devastates an engineer.

"Doc, I assume that you do not believe in botanicals".

"That is right. I would not muddy the waters now. Let's see what happens after we stop the TPN."

Dr. Broth then departed in a jolly mood leaving with some words of encouragement. The TPN was stopped immediately. Nevertheless the liver enzymes shot up further the next day. Dr. Broth came by again.

"Doc, what do you think?"

"The enzymes went up, it does not look good."

"I need to ask you again about some botanicals. Do you know of any?"

"I know them all!

"What about some alpha lipoic acid?"

"Well, it is not going to hurt or help."

"Then you are not opposed if I administer some."

"Not at all."

After my conversation with the liver specialist, I gave Elizabeth some lipoic acid, and the next day the enzymes made a reversal. Elizabeth kept vomiting blood, did not eat and became progressively weaker. On March 5 Dr. Newmade said, "We need to give her a steroid drug called Decadron. It should relieve her vomiting in about a day."

There followed some back and forth and the final conversation about Decadron follows.

"Doc, this Decadron is counter-indicated in case of a fungal infection."

"She does not have a fungal infection and I cannot discuss this any further. I am tired, and if you wish I can cancel it."

"No, go ahead if this is your best judgment."

I refrained from asking, "What the hell was that Fluconasole for if she did not have a fungal infection?" Elizabeth got two infusions of Decadron. She started shaking so violently that they stopped it immediately. The next day they came to me with Prilosec and Marinol. Now, Prilosec can kill a healthy liver. Elizabeth's remnants of a liver were just enough for her to hang on.

"That is a NO!"

"But, the attending doctor Dr. Strident, ordered it!"

"Then this is a resounding NO!

"Brainless application of double-edged pharmaceuticals."

That is all I could think at the moment.

Throughout all these twelve days, the Prince was out of sight. He was "attending" during February, which meant that he was in charge on the floor. We saw him during the rounds in the morning with a group of residents and students or whatever, typical for a teaching hospital. I kept hoping that he would stop by for a talk about Elizabeth. There was a lot to discuss, an assessment of the situation, were there any measures other than those standards being constantly looked up in the fat pharmaceutical handbooks by his young, mostly female residents? What would he do after the recovery? The chemos seemed to be exhausted. Would he help to get Elizabeth into some biologicals trials? Most importantly, I badly needed help from him with my mental turmoil: Should I stop making these extraordinary efforts to rescue her from the present crisis, especially the liver crisis? If I did, would I set her up for the inevitable cancer pain? Would I be doing her a terrible disservice by not letting her slide away now? I had been told that liver failure was a relatively painless process. "She will get disoriented and confused and slide into a coma, she will not know what is happening," said Doctor Broth. To rescue her would make great sense if she would participate further in the fight for her life, go back fully to our "Contra Program" and extend viability as long as possible. Maybe in the meantime, she could win the Monoclonal Antibody (a novel less toxic biological treatment) Lottery; maybe some new development would come along. With her mental exhaustion and her always negative and intransigent attitude her recovery from the present crisis might mean horrible suffering in the near future. Was all that reasoning correct in light of her condition? Even if it was correct, could I withhold what I knew could help her temporarily now? The Prince never stopped by to help me with my agony. On his last attending day, February 28, he sat at the desk and busily wrote reports. I pretended often, to go to the restroom so that he could see me. He left the floor and did not stop by, nor the next day or the day after. Not even after the intensive care crisis. Not when Elizabeth's liver situation became so critical. Why did I not approach him directly that time? Because I knew he could help little with the immediate crisis. He was an oncologist and Elizabeth's problems were not in his line, he had "specialists." What I needed was his humanity more than his medical input into my excruciating personal dilemmas.

These were my bitter thoughts during the long hours waiting for the Prince, who never came: "Dr. Hope, I do not want to face you ever again. You have betrayed my high faith in you. You deserted me in the darkest hour of my struggle and I even wonder if you are man enough to understand what I have just said." These were my thoughts at the time.

Elizabeth came home on Saturday, March 7. Initially, things did not look too bad. The trouble started in the evening of that day. She had to go to the bathroom every hour or so, but could not get up by herself. Even with my trying to support her with all my strength she kept collapsing on the floor and I had to leave her there, arranging a makeshift bed in front of the bathroom door. Her eyes rolled in distress; she often asked, "Where am I?" She started to have all kinds of weird sensations like "ears hot and burning". She desperately tried to maintain some dignity with the restroom problem. This situation kept worsening by the hour until Sunday mid–morning, when she lay on the floor half-conscious. We called an ambulance.

The rest of Sunday was agony. She started bleeding from the mouth and rectum. She suffered terribly most of the afternoon in the intensive care unit until a steadily increasing dose of morphine took effect. Our son Jack and I stroked her hands and arms, Jack and I on either side. I watched her struggling for air despite the oxygen mask, her breast heaving in deep strokes that became less and less frequent. She looked at me with a strange expression. Only after days had passed could I venture a guess as to what it was. It must have been the last spiteful curiosity,

"You can see that I am dying, how does it feel to you?"

After an hour of her not responding, her breathing became less frequent but still very heavy and labored. This went on for another hour, her heart not giving up. The doctor said, "The oxygen keeps her heart pumping, should we take it away?"

"Yes."

On the monitor, we could see her heart slowing down steadily until it stopped. I asked to be alone with her for a few minutes. I was close to fainting but managed to whisper "Good bye, my love" into her ear. I placed my last kiss on her now calm and not yet cold forehead.

This was the eighth of March, 7.30 PM, 1998, two months short of three years from the time of the first diagnosis. In July Elizabeth would have been 62.

So, by the thoughtless application of protocols and without an effort at "intellectualizing" they had shortened Elizabeth's life, by how much? Nobody can answer that question. God only knows how shabby most doctors are in light of the fact that we dealt with one of unusual attentiveness (at times) and ability.

This horrible story has come to its conclusion. No more facts or information are going to come in. The doctor–patient relationship has come to an end. It is time to look back and assess coolly my relationship with Dr. Hope. In a synthesis of all that has happened, I would say to Dr. Hope: "You have had and do have our appreciation. We are grateful for the periods when you showed interest and humanity, for the time and understanding you have given me in my effort to help, and the attention given to Elizabeth. You are an extraordinary doctor considering what the entire lot appears to be. Your dedication to your profession is exceptional, not usually seen with other doctors. I myself have witnessed the long hours and the weekends away from your family. I would implore you to reflect upon what I have written. You are a professor of medicine. Your patients expect extraordinary feats from you, and these can be only accomplished by persistent and dogged pursuit, often outside the "party line." You are their last hope in this life. It was Elizabeth's last wish and my fervent and still living wish that you break out of protocols, and the arcane code of behavior, in the establishment – this is so destructive. Use your own judgment, damn the coordinators, and broaden your vision. Become a true Prince of medicine, break out, and break out!"

Closing Remarks

The history of Elizabeth's illness demonstrates the "rot" present in the medical profession; (I reluctantly use this term, profession, for lack of a more appropriate one). It is an organization protected by and in collusion with the government bureaucracy. It protects itself from scrutiny and is not responsible to anyone. In any true profession that serves the needs of people, mistakes are mostly aired or become obvious, the honest ones understood and forgiven, the ones committed out of callousness or negligence are punished one way or another, but not in medicine. There, mutual protection and obfuscation will bury anything, except exceptional foul–ups, such as amputating the wrong leg. The public, being a captive population, has nowhere else to turn. Helpless, we mill around trying in desperation to find some practitioner with a human face who might be professional. There is no competition except the budding alternative sector, which does not have the resources or technology and is harassed by the government.

As with any monopoly, they do what they please with impunity under the protection of the state. It also strikes me that the individual doctor is not accountable to anyone for his professional actions. He has no boss to oversee him, to report on his actions or evaluate his results. It is not possible to pose questions after one dies, and the family members left behind are usually so befuddled and ignorant of what really has happened that they accept explanations at face value. This is quite a unique situation in the professional world, when the rest of us have our bosses to please. It keeps us on our toes in a constant state of alertness and responsibility. These guys have but one concern – protecting their own turf.

Do I have anything good to say? Oh... yes. The technical side is superb. Here are the words of a transplant surgeon whom I befriended at UCLA. He was exposed to his own kind when he waited for a liver transplant for his wife.

"The one who treated Mary was impossible to see without an appointment made 4-6 weeks in advance. He is always traveling and taking pictures with his 35 mm. In fact, I wonder which is his vocation and which his avocation. Mary was treated by protocol and I really do not think that he did much intellectualization about her problem. *On the other hand, the technicians - here I'm*

*not using it as a pejorative word - the invasive radiologist
who put the catheter into the liver going to the tumor
and the surgeon performing the transplant, were
magnificently proficient"*. [An irony – in light of the
above our Prince is superb! S.S.]

The machinery for diagnostics is fabulous and
the facilities are generally the best in the world. The
laboratories for blood and other diagnostic work are
superb. The nursing staff is professional and caring.
Only when the **High Priests of the Cabal** enter the
scene does one get a sinking feeling of doubt, concern
and frustration. These haughty fellows are callous, they
do not think, they are arrogant and dismissive, they do
not care to explore and investigate, they blindly follow
protocols and they think that dying is not a big deal at
all. The patient should die when told to do so; otherwise
the situation becomes unsettling and burdensome.
Damn those husband activists who do not let their
wives die by protocol!

From the above generalization, one can find
exceptions, but these exceptions are still troubling. Let's
take Dr. Alternate. He, without doubt, prolonged
Elizabeth's life by unorthodox thinking, by caring and
by being his own master, and not looking over his

shoulder to the COORDINATOR. But there it stops. He would not bring himself to call our doctor to discuss our case or to advise him of a possible approach because according to the medical etiquette this could be perceived as interference. Etiquette over lives!

Etiquette! The medical practitioners in the system of official medicine are bound by a set of unspoken and arcane conventions. They will never criticize a colleague, or intervene in the slightest to point out even an obvious mistake about to happen. Added to this is an equally complex set of official dos and don'ts. Mix into this the fear of lawsuits and we end up with a system where it is difficult to find independent thinking from inquisitive doctors who would doggedly go after a solution, outside the established canons if necessary. That is a basic demand put on other professions. In short, we have a callous, mechanical and calcified system of prescribed motions. *__It hasn't been approved yet__*, is often the answer to questions about a novel approach.

Sven Sonnenberg

North Carolina, Fall 1998

Alternative Measures

Most people are oblivious to medical matters. Very often, they have poor knowledge in basics of nutrition, personal hygiene, and environmental influences on their health. Sometimes, even with a rudimentary awareness of harmful habits they still smoke or indulge in unhealthy habits like excessive alcohol consumption et cetera.

When a health disaster strikes, the obvious place to turn to is the medical establishment. It would not enter anybody's mind to ignore the establishment and seek alternative measures as their first choice. Even for people who are somewhat cognizant of the role of nutrition and the existence of a vast alternative movement in health matters, it is excruciatingly difficult for them to make health decisions by themselves, or for their loved ones. For the untrained, it seems presumptuous and irresponsible to choose a course of action not sanctioned by the official medicine, the FDA, et cetera et cetera. The most frequent reaction I got from my friends was, "I could never take the responsibility and do what you are doing."

So, what does one do? The first look at the alternative landscape is overwhelming. There is a multitude of organizations, doctors, clinics, that claim miracles and warn of going with the beaten path of the official medicine. Unfortunately, if one starts to investigate, then one finds that it is almost impossible to verify the claims with any independent reviews or even with data published by this or that organization. The so-called anecdotal reports abound. Where does one turn to? If one forgoes chemotherapy, radiation and surgery, would this be a foolhardy decision, a sure death sentence? Well, there is one report to turn to first. It is the

"Unconventional Cancer Treatments" Published by the Office of Technology assessment- US Department of Commerce.

There, at least, there is an attempt to investigate impartially. The unfortunate situation is that this Government Entity is unable to show or supply convincing evidence that this or that treatment works most of the time. And here comes the rub. If the diagnosis rendered is a hopeful one—localized cancer, possible to treat by excision with some follow up treatment, then the attention to alternative measures should go only as far as improving the overall health status, Vitamin, mineral supplementation, changes in **lifestyle** along guidelines of some alternative practitioners.

What if the diagnosis is: **"Three months to live, we can do little."** Well, what does one do then? That is where a number of people say, "Nothing to lose" and an intense search for an alternative approach should begin. The problem then is what to choose and where to go. The choices are overwhelming — excruciating to consider. It seems that the choices are like playing the lottery. There are however, some institutions and some practitioners who have something of a record of accomplishment and are in "business" for a considerable time. I will list them in order of my own "whim", or let's say estimate. Many can show anecdotal successes not verified by an independent agency or governmental entity, nevertheless these are difficult to ignore.

I will enclose here an excerpt from the writings of Dr. Douglas Campbell. It is harsh, but to add weight to what he has to say one must remember that in case of a metastasis condition the very doctor who rushes the patient to chemotherapy says outright, "There is no hope for a cure."

He puts the patient trough an agony of side effects and it is truly a matter of what will kill the patient first the cancer or chemotherapy. In the case, just described two things are clear. Eventually at the end of chemotherapy, the oncologists have killed Elizabeth, after inflicting severe suffering, fortunately during a very brief period at the end. The other point is also clear, that without the alternative support, which mitigated the effects of the chemotherapy and prolonged her life and gave her a reasonable quality of life Elizabeth would go through debilitating suffering all along without the hope of a cure, like many of her co-patients in the clinic. The "establishment" oncologist admitted that much. I had a case where a friend's wife was in Elizabeth's condition. He asked me for my program, but she refused to do anything other than her doctors ordered. She was dead in six months after suffering all the debilitating effects of the treatment they (the doctors) administered.

Here is Dr. Campbell's take:

Oncologists- "Jackals among men"

If there is any medical treatment that ranks down there with psychotherapy as quack medicine, it is chemotherapy. Although it can be helpful in cases of testicular cancer and lymphocytic leukemia, chemotherapy is basically fraudulent and illogical. How in the world can oncologists think they are treating rationally when their so-called therapy is destroying the immune system?

Sure, the tumor may shrink-because its immunity is being attacked as well. So it becomes a race as to which will kill the patient first: the cancer or the treatment? Yet, oncologists are so fanatical that they say chemotherapy should be employed EVEN IF WE KNOW IT DOESN'T WORK! One leading oncologist remarked that "chemotherapy serves an extremely valuable role in keeping patients oriented toward proper medical therapy .... Judicious employment and screening of potentially useful

drugs may also prevent the spread of cancer quackery". This is a preposterous statement. Treating a patient with advanced cancer with toxic drugs that you know will not work, and will increase the suffering of the patient, is the essence of quackery.

Even the doctors know there's no cure.

When asked why patients never hear the "C" word and are told instead, "You have a tumor, " the author of a book on disease disclosure said that deception is necessary so that patients will not "begin hunting about for that will-o -the-wisp that is a cancer cure. " So, you see, the doctors have given up on a cure for cancer. They know their drugs are often worse than useless but feel they must be given any way to keep patients out of the hands of "a charlatan who promises results while he impoverishes the family. " Well, how is this for impoverishing the family? A course of fosfamide, one of mainstream medicine's killer drugs, costs (in 1995) $10,000 for a five-day course. And that's only for the drug and so does not include the doctor's fee, all the hospital costs, and he costs of treating the *horrible side effects. Not to mention that there are usually two other expensive drugs prescribed at the same time. All this can easily run up a bill of a million dollars. That's just a sum to keep a quack from "impoverishing the family".*

To better understand the utter hypocrisy of chemotherapy, consider the following: The McGill Cancer Center in Canada, one of the largest and most prestigious cancer treatment centers in the world, did a study of oncologists to determine how they would respond to a diagnosis of cancer. On the confidential questionnaire, 58 out of 64 doctors said that all chemotherapy programs were unacceptable to them and their family members. The overriding reason for this decision was that the drugs are ineffective and have an unacceptable degree of toxicity. These are the same doctors who will tell you that their chemotherapy treatments will shrink your tumor and prolong your life!

It takes one to know one.

Oncologist James Holland once stated: *"My definition of cancer quackery is the deliberate misapplication of a diagnostic or treatment procedure in a patient with cancer .... The culprit who victimizes his fellow man suffering from cancer ... all the while greedily enriching himself, is a quack, a criminal, a jackal among men who deserves the scorn and ostracism of society. Because human life is at stake, he must be controlled.* "Of course, Dr. Holland is not referring to his colleagues and himself but instead to all other doctors offering alternatives to the ferociously toxic chemotherapy drugs. Certainly, there are quacks in the alternative cancer-treatment field. But by Dr. Holland's own definition, every oncologist is a quack.

Thirty years ago, I worked with a radiologist who told me this: "I get cancer; I'm going to Mexico". So if you get cancer, don't call your doctor; call your travel agent.

Action to take:
There are alternative treatments available, but you will have to run the gamut of outraged chemotherapists, radiologists, and surgeons to find one. They will use cajolery, insults, fear, threats ("If

you do this, I am off the case"), and misrepresentation to dissuade you.

Two excellent clinics offering alternative treatments are the following: -Burton Clinic in the Bahamas P.O. Box 42689

- *Freeport, Grand Bahamas Island*
Tel. (242)352-7455, Fax (242)352-3201, www.iatclinic.com

- *Burzynski Clinic in Houston, TX 9432 Old Katy Rd.*
Houston, TX 77055
Tel. (713)335-5697, Fax (713)335-5699, www.cancermed.com

   Also, doctors affiliated with The American College for Advancement in Medicine may be able to provide a promising therapy called photochemotherapy-in which a small portion (a glassful) of blood is withdrawn from the patient's vein, exposed to ultraviolet light and then injected back into the patient's body.

Read ,Questioning Chemotherapy, by Ralph Moss,

Equinox Press. This book is a must for all concerned about this medical scandal-a chamber of horrors that doctors don't want to talk about."

The above excerpt is an opinion of an experienced doctor. It is seconded by many others often not in such condemning terms, nevertheless pointing out the problems with the officially approved mainstream medical establishment and their methods.

There is plenty of writing declaring all the so-called alternative programs quackery. These papers are often written by mainstream doctors with such vehemence and condemnation that one gets suspicious right away of their motives and truthfulness. Difficult indeed is for the patient to find his way through this dangerous maze. For balance, I will cite here an Internet address of a site that purports to debunk of all that quackery.

http://www.quackwatch.org/01QuackeryRelatedTopic s/cancer.html Dr. Steven Barett, a psychiatrist, operates that site. He also edits a book titled: *"Vitamins and Minerals: Help or Harm." "While some questionable therapies are harmless or inexpensive, others have toxic effects and may be costly, and none have scientifically proven efficacy."*

The above is their summary statement. The problem with these people is that they will not even acknowledge the importance but often condemn the use of nutrition and supplementation, as was the case for us at that World Renowned Cancer Center.

Following, I will list places that seem to give some hope of not being just "quackery." These will be the places to begin the search and to contact and explore. One has to remember that the choice has to be based on the type of cancer and the condition the patient is in. For example: The Burzynski Institute's strength is in brain tumors.

Read the "Unconventional Cancer Treatments."
Publication PB91-104 893,
Office of technology Assessment, Washington, DC
U.S department of Commerce tel. 1-888584 8332
Consult to find a good doctor for your case:

"Best Doctors in America" Phone 1- 800- 675-1199
 E-mail cgreamee@bestdoctors.com
Their web site: www.bestdoctors.com

Their Motto is:

No one has got the last word.

There is all kinds of information out there and you've got to take the initiative to find it.

Under this title, I have to list Dr. Suzan Love. She is heading The Susan Love Research Foundation. Her web site is: http://www.dslrf.org

It is important to read Suzanne Somers book **"Knock Out, Interviews with doctors who are CURING CANCER."**

I will cite a critical excerpt from an interview with Dr. Forsythe,

...You know, Susan, it's much easier to be a conventional oncologist, because you just tell the patient to be in the transfusion center on Monday and the protocol is recommended. We give them their dose schedule and we do not deviate. As an oncologist doing it this way, you'll never get in trouble even if the patient dies from your treatment. But if you go outside the box at all and add vitamins or anything

alternative, that's when the criticism comes down on you...

And another important statement:

"...Because I am a conventional board-certified oncologist, I offer conventional protocol chemo first. Basically, I do that because of its legality. I am required by law to offer "standard care". I once had an FDA agent tell me that I was depriving patients of the benefit of conventional chemo, and I kind of had to laugh under my breath at that..."

Alternative Cancer Centers:

There is such a multitude of Alternative Cancer Centers in the USA and abroad, especially in Mexico that it is almost impossible to list all of them much less to recommend on a basis of proved records. The few listed below have gained wider publicity and can show some results.

1. **D. James Forsythe**
Century Wellness Clinic

http://www.drforsythe.com/
Century Wellness Clinic 521
Hammill Lane Reno, NV 89511-1004
(775) 827-0707

2. Block Medical Center

Comprehensive Health Services

1800 SHERMAN AVENUE SUITE 515

EVANSTON, IL 60201

708-492-3040, FAX 708- 492-3045

http://www.blockmd.com/

3. Burzynski Clinic in Houston, TX

9432 Old Katy Rd.

Houston, TX 77055

Tel. (713) 335-5697, Fax (713)335-5699

www.cancermed.com

4. ITL Cancer Clinic (Bahamas) Ltd. P.O. Box F-42689, Freeport, Grand Bahama, Bahamas. (877) 785-

http://immunemedicine.com/

Phone: (242) 352-7455

Fax: (242) 352-3201

mail@immunemedicine.com

Below is a comment concerning IAT (ITL) and the Burton Method. However, the above Clinic offers an array of other methods, many listed in the Alternative arsenal.

IAT is claimed to have about a 19% effectiveness rate. Various cancers respond differently to IAT:

As of this writing, no one claims that IAT cures cancer. Proponents claim that the therapy can stop the spread of many cancers and may send the cancer into remission. They claim that by treating deficiencies or imbalances in the immune system, the body is able treat itself, resulting in an extended lifespan and enhanced quality of life. Sometimes the disease has spread too far within the body to respond to IAT. Furthermore, if chemotherapy or radiation treatment has over-suppressed the immune system, response to IAT may be slow.

5. Nicholas Gonzalez, M.D.

36 at East 36th St, Suite 204

New York, NY, 1001

Tel: 212-213-3337or fax----3414

http://www.dr-gonzalez.com/

The National Cancer Institute (NCI) has sponsored a study to evaluate the nutritional treatment of pancreatic cancer at his clinic. That trial apparently running years and stopped has a rich literature form many corners including Dr. Gonzalez. Before commuting one should read, and begin with:

http://www.sciencebasedmedicine.org/index.php/the-gonzalez-trial-for-pancreatic-cancer-outcome-revealed/.

This clinic is written up in Burton Goldberg's book. "An alternative medicine definitive guide to cancer."

http://www.burtongoldberg.com/consultations. Unfortunately the cruel expression used after a jury awarded a penalty against Dr. Gonzalez's Center (Operating in New York) for a death of a lady's husband is:

"In other words, social Darwinism, (i.e., people

unable to spot a quack deserve whatever they get) rules."

COLEY'S TOXIN

An immunological approach

There is one alternate therapy, which has fallen into obscurity for quite a long time, because of the emergence of Chemotherapy and other treatments. Now it is undergoing a revival and there is activity on that subject which broadly is termed immunological treatment. The champion of this approach is Dr. Lloyd I. Old, M.D. of Ludwig Institute for Cancer Research New York, New York and Ms. Helen Coley-Nauts at the Cancer Research Institute

http://www.cancerresearch.org/

There is a very informative blog under http://cancerwife.com/ the first article to read is Coley's Toxins Introduction and a personal story, titled:

"Why Coley's Toxins has not been widely used despite its results."

The Waisbren Clinic in Milwaukee, Wisconsin, treats patients with cancer with a mixed bacterial vaccine consisting of modified Coley toxins plus 10 strains of the heat killed streptococcus bacteria which causes burn infections, plus BCG, transfer factor donated by relatives of patients, and a strain of lymphoblastoid lymphocytes combined with Epstein-Barr virus [20]. An uncontrolled clinical series study by that center is reviewed within the Summary of Research and Annotated Bibliographic sections of this therapy review. Further information concerning the treatment at that clinic is available at that web site[21].

http://www.waisbrenclinic.com/

Dr. Moerman's Anti-Cancer Diet

While searching around the world, I came across Dr. Moerman who practiced in Holland for almost half a century. He had some successes and the insurances in Holland accepted his treatment as legitimate. However, in advanced cancer cases his treatment was much less effective. Therefore, the alternative practitioners did not recommend Dr. Moerman's approach. However, I found some merits in his recommendations and support for some of his compounds in other publications. These were Iodine and sulfur. I have included it in Elizabeth's table of Vitamins and Minerals. There is a note there referring how to prepare the Iodine and it is:

> Iodine - 3 tablespoon solution daily - 1 tablespoon three times daily (Iodii spirit, 3%. Mix 1 to 3 drops in 300 g. water or red sour wine) - "This can be prepared using equal parts of the iodii spirit and the other liquid, depending on the severity of the case" - found in iodized salt, which is not allowed on this diet, thus it must be supplemented.

Other supplemental and dietary recommendation can be found in:

http://www.cancertutor.com/Cancer/Moerman.html

There is a huge body of literature about cancer. Obviously, mainstream, medicine has massive volumes, some of which I have studied and were in use by Elizabeth's doctor. I will list those in references.

There are also a number of shorter publications with definite claims. I will list a few as an example of that category. It is doubtful if one ought to jump into some of those methods advocated. These publications mostly give as a support testimonials of people supposedly cured. It is my guess that some individual cases could be true, but they are probably exceptions. I will cite here Dr. Forsythe again *... **But individual case studies hold no credence. No conventional oncologist would take an individual case seriously...***

Unless, I need to add quickly, when the official/conventional medicine has given up, or concludes, "NOTHING CAN BE DONE SHE HAS THREE MONTHS AT THE MOST." AND THE PATIENT TAKES MATTERS INTO HIS OR HER OWN HANDS.

Therefore, it is necessary to investigate records of accomplishment, history and proven results as much as possible.

1. "Natural Cancer Remedies that Work". Morton Walker D.P.M published by Finn Communications

2. "Cancer Defeated!" by Frank, COUSINEAU

Andrew Scholberg- Online Publishing &
Marketing LLC.

3. German Cancer Breakthrough, by Andrew
Scholberg

4. Cancer Breakthrough USA, by Frank COUSINEAU
with Andrew Scholberg

5. Ultimate Cancer Breakthrough by Aparajita
&Marko Wutzer

In most cases the patient is not in a mental
condition to conduct such an investigation. A close
friend or relative (the husband) should, therefore,
become competent in research. It is of crucial
importance to assist, and time usually is of essence! The
problem here is one of patient participation and
decisions should ultimately rest with him or her. It is
excruciatingly difficult and sometimes impossible to
push one's spouse into this or that treatment especially
when going away from the mainstream medicine. This
was my problem and I chose a compromise. Who can
tell if I was right? Even today, after so much time has

elapsed and after extensive study, I do not know!

To give you a glimpse of what one faces I will discuss one recommendation out of the booklets with the title BREAKTHROUGH!

From Frank COUSINEAU's booklet, the **"Cancer Treatment of America"**

http://www.cancercenter.com/

Reading the reports of patients and their experiences one's head goes into a dizzy rotation. Their advertisements promise the sky, but a good percentage of reports are dismal. "Money grabbing machine with incompetent doctors, or rather actors, with no idea about medicine." There is a fair amount of good experiences depending on the center location - Philly or Arizona et cetera. What caught my eye was a piece by a professional reporter—not by a patient. In effect, he said he could recognize the positive reports as written by the Center under the patient's name. "Hey"... he says, "be human, make some spelling mistakes in your blog piece."

So, what should the husband DO?

In the last chapter you will read what husbands do. Some RUN. I for one did not run and took more than a burden, but still I am hesitant to blame those who do run. However, the least you can do is give the best comfort to your spouse, but that may be too little. Of course, if you have a recalcitrant wife who does not want to fight and goes with the "official" flow and you feel you are competent to help, then it is a torturous situation. In a word, it is HELL.

Elizabeth's Program

A. Vitamins and Minerals

B. Dietary Points, for Elizabeth

C. Other Important Points

D. One of Elizabeth's Diet Days

Elizbeth's VITMINS AND MINERALS

COMPOUND	DOSE	#/DAY	1	2	3	4	5	6	
Times Approx.			8:00 AM	10:30am	1:00AM	4:30 PM	7:30 PM	10:30 PM	
GARLIC (KYOLIC)	2 CAPS	3	X		X		X		
VITAMIN C with BIOFLAVONOIDS	3000 mg	6	X	X	X	X	X	X	
VITAMIN A	10,000 mg	2	X			X			
VITAMIN D3	400 mg	2	X			X			Watch serum CALCIUM
BETA-CAROTENE	25,000 mg	5	X	X	X	X	X	X	
VITAMIN E	400 IU	3	X		X		X		
SELENIUM	100 mcg	5	X	X	X	X	X		
VITAMIN B COMPLEX B1 B2 Niacinamide B6 B12 Folic Acid Biotin Pantotheic Acid	TAB 50 mg 50 mg 50mg 50mg 50mg 400mcg 50mg 50mg	2	X			X			
FOLIC ACID	800 mcg	1				X			
SOD	2000	2	X			X			
CITRIC ACID	1 tblsp	3	X		X		X		Very Important: see Dr. Moerman in the Altertnative section to prepare solution. Improper use is harmfull
IODINE	1 tblsp	3	X		X		X		
SULPHUR	500 mg	2	X				X		
GLUTADIONE	50 mg	2		X		X			
Q10 ENZIME	100 mg	3	X		X		X		increase to 4/day
MAGNEZIUM	250 mg	2		X			X		
ZINC	50 mg	1					X		
GRAPE SEED (PYCNOGENOL PHYTOSOME)	50 mg	2		X		X			
ESSIAC - HERBAL	2 oz	2	X VERY IMPORTANT: CAN USE ALSO FLORE-ESSENCE, BUT CAUTION WITH ESTROGEN POSITIVE RECEPTOR CANCERS< TALK TO YOUR DOC/TOR/ONCOLOGIST					X	

ELIZABETH'S VITAMINS AND MINERALS								
KELP		2	X					X
PROBIOTIC CULTURES (ACIDOPHILUS +OTHERS)	210mg	3	X		X			X
L- CYSTEINE	500mg	1		X				
L-METHIONINE	500mg	1				X		
L-ORNITHINE	500mg	1						X
L-LYSINE	500mg					X		
WHEAT GRASS	350mg	6	X	X	X	X	X	X
CALCIUM	500mg	2		X		X	Calcium /Magnesium/ D Vit. complex	
COPPER	2mg	Every Other Day			X			
THYMUS	185mg	3	X		X		X	
B-6 *in addition to multi B*	100mg			X				X
Molybdenum Chelated	300 mg	1				X		

Note: Pay attention to sequence. Egzample:
Selenium generally with Vitamin E, Zinc not with Calcium. Eat something before bedtime to combine with last pills.

NOTE: A NUTRITIONAL PROFILE WAS DONE AT DIFFERENT TIMES OF THE TREATMENT CYCLE AND ADJUSTMENTS UP OR DOWN OR ADDITION SHOULD BE MADE TO THE ABOVE LIST . ONE OF POSSIBLE SERVICES IS: Metametrix Clinical Laboratory
3425 Corporate Way Duluth, GA 30096 USA (800) 221-4640, (770) 446-5483

B. Instructions for Elizabeth

Dietary Points

- **Limit dairy products. Use yogurt, kefir. Cut out cheeses. Limit milk- use only low fat, skimmed or 1%.**

    Organic eggs

- **No animal fat, limit meat**

    Limit coffee

    No alcohol

    No refined sugar

No margarines, poly or saturated oils. Use extra virgin olive oil only, For seasoning you can use some flavoring oils like sesame or others but sparingly.

- **Drink green tea as a main drink throughout the day**

- **As main staples use whole grain breads**

    Brown rice, beans, soybeans especially

    Whole wheat grains pastas, noodles

    Grain of all sorts, barley etc.

    Peas, soybean products - tofu etc.

    Shitake Mushrooms

- Raw vegetables, tomatoes, cucumbers. Make salads. Use romaine lettuce and a lot of other greens.

  Steamed not cooked vegetables for dinners, especially Brussels sprouts, broccoli and cabbage.

- Generous amounts of fruits eaten raw, especially oranges, grapefruit and other citruses.

- Juices, as many glasses as you can. No less than 2 glasses of carrot mixed with red beet and one lemon.

- 8 ounces or more of deep sea fish a week (salmon or others)

- Lemons at every turn and into everywhere you can - salad dressings, into juices etc.

- Garlic, use garlic as much as you can. Add to salad dressing, to sauces made with stewed tomato in olive oil and onions and so on. Garlic at every turn, it contains Germanium - very important

- In general, avoid:

- **Processed Foods**

  Refined flour, sugars

  Hydrogenated oils

  Animal fats & products

  Canned foods

  Cereals with hydrogenated oils and chemicals

- **Buy organically grown food where possible and feasible , especially when liver decease is present.**

- **Buy and read the following books, at least!**

Find your type of cancer	1. CANCER THERAPY
	the independent consumer
Use as many compounds	
	To non-toxic treatments
as you can from the table in the	
	by Ralph W. Moss,
guide at the beginning of the book	EQUINOX PRESS
and combine instructions with those of No. 1 and No. 2	

Note how much discipline

It takes to succeed

2.Cancer
Battle Plan
Anne E.
Frahm , David
J. Frahm
PINON PRESS

3. Prescription for
Nutritional Healing.
James f. Balch,
Phyllis A. Balch
AVERY PUBLISH-
ING GROUP

Read 3 Papers by Dr. Keith Block

1. Dietary Impact on Quality of life in Cancer

2. Dietary change in lifestyle Factors in Patients

Surviving Advanced Malignancies

3. Nutrition: An essential tool in Cancer Therapy

Obtain Papers from The Block Center

5230 Old Orchard Road Skokie, IL 60077

1-877-41-BLOCK (1-877-412-5625) --

C. OTHER IMPORTANT NOTES

- Exercise! The more the better. Run, use machines. Discipline yourself to put in an equivalent of 3 miles of a brisk walk every day.

- For nausea during chemotherapy use ginger root tablets instead of the standard pharmaceutical. Do not use tap water for cooking and drinking, buy bottled spring water.

- Rinse your mouth with salt water during chemotherapy to avoid sores

- Be careful with prescription drugs—avoid using if you can, try to find alternative natural remedies as above.

- Carefully monitor your clinic or hospital treatment, ask for blood test results (especially white cell count) keep your own record, read, and learn the meaning of other tests. Prepare questions for your doctor. Request meetings. Do not allow yourself to be brushed off with un-thoughtful answers, see if you can come up with some of your own ideas for tests or alternative approaches.

- Read, Read, Read!

D. One of Elizabeth's Diet Days

8.00 Am Large Bowl of fruits

- 1 orange or grapefruit
- 1 banana
- 1 apple
- 4-5 strawberries
- juice from 1 lemon

  put all above in blender, eat all at once or trough morning

11.00 AM Yogurt and cereal

- Nonfat yogurt, Stonyfield Farm, add raw crushed almonds
- any cereal organic without hydrogenated fats and sugar

2.00 PM   **Salad with dressing**

Bread whole wheat spread with tahini

Salad - green salad, tomatoes,

peppers cucumbers

Dressing - olive oil, garlic, lemon juice

5.00 PM **Juice** from 3 carrots, 1 lemon, small red beet

7.30 - 8.00 PM **Dinner**

Alternate with some meat and fish dishes

- soup, steamed vegetables with extra virgin olive oil + 1 - lemon juice

- whole wheat pasta with sauce, or brown rice with sauce

    sauce is prepared from

-     tomatoes
-     chopped onions
-     green peppers
-     maitake and shitake mushrooms
-     all stewed in olive oil

10.30 - 11.00 PM **Fruit snack** to get the last pills down

8.00 am, 11.00 am and 5.00 pm is almost always fixed, 2.00 PM and dinner is varied, including beans in a variety on type and preparation. 2 times a week we have fish 4 ounces each time, broiled with rice and steamed vegetables. For desert typically we have home baked banana bread or ginger bread

5. References

1."Cancer of the Breast" William L. Donegan M.D. FACS, John S. Spratt M.D. FACS

2. Clinical Oncology Philip Rubin M.D.

3. Susan Love,s Breast Book, Susan M. Love M.D.

4. Cancer Free, Sidney j. Winawer M.D. Moshe

   Shike M.D. Both at Memorial Sloan_Kettering

   Cancer Center

5. "Unconventional Cancer Treatments".

Publication PB91-104 893,

Office of technology Assessment, Washington, DC

   US department of Commerce tel. 1-888584r.

6. Cancer Therapy, Ralph W. Moss PhD

7. Dr. Keith Block, Block Medical Center,

Evanston, IL

   a. Dietary Impact on Quality of life in Cancer

   b. Dietary change in lifestyle Factors in

      Patients

   Surviving Advanced Malignancies

   c. Nutrition: An essential tool in Cancer

   Therapy

8. Dietary Antioxidants during Cancer

Chemotherapy: Impact on Chemotherapeutic

Effectiveness and Development of side
effects. Kenneth A. Conklin M.D. in
Nutrition
And Cancer 2000, 37(1), 1-18

9. The Savage Cell, Pat McGrady

10. Numerous Magazine publications, among
others
Current Opinion in ONCOLOGY, a
bimonthly, Rapid Science Publisher

Information on Comprehensive Cancer Treatment Centers

I have selected places to begin the search:

Cancer Control Society

http://www.nccn.org/members/network.asp

http://cancercontrolsociety.com

There are about 9,740,000 entries on the Internet under the key phrase "Comprehensive Cancer Treatment." Comprehensive probably means that there is the basics plus a full array of additional capabilities including extensive technology, counseling, hospital, and sometimes nutritional counseling. The first inclination is to go to the nearest center that offers cancer treatment. This perhaps is not the wisest decision. A probing research is needed of where to really start treatment. The diagnosing family doctor will probably send the patient to what he/she thinks is the most convenient and sometimes to the one he/she is associated with. That happened with us, but we immediately went to a renowned, world famous institution for a second opinion and to explore the facility. We did not like it and as time proceeded, we were glad that we stayed with the original, where our doctor sent us. And even there, we were lucky to encounter an unusual and caring doctor, different than the rest in that place. It is important to have an individual connection with the particular doctor, so that one can talk to him, know that he is paying attention, is open to discussion, is going to help with your exploration and will stand by you when you explore alternatives. It was clear to us from the outset that in that World Renowned Institution we would not be listened to; it would be their arrogant way, period. That often happens with large famous outfits. They become arrogant and uncaring and the patient becomes a number. Did they have something special? Oh... no, just the general protocols approved by the ECOG tsar of the:

Eastern Cooperative Oncology Group (ECOG).

Perhaps a good example is melanoma. In that case, one can find many places for treatment. However, there is one pioneering place to explore and it is:

Steven A. Rosenberg, M.D., Ph.D.

Surgery Branch

Head, Tumor Immunology Section

Branch Chief

Building 10-CRC, Room 3-3940

10 Center Drive, MSC 1201

Bethesda, MD 20892

Phone:

301-496-4164

Fax:

301-402-1738

E-Mail:

SAR@nih.gov

The trick then is to be able to qualify for his programs. We inquired for Elizabeth, but the answer was "Sorry, we have nothing for breast cancer." A good example how much exploration is needed.

CANCER

NEW CHEMICAL MARKERS WILL TAILOR THE TREATMENT TO THE DISEASE

REGIONS ■ Northeast ■ South ■ West ■ Midwest

Rank	Hospital	U.S. News Score	Reputation (%)	Mortality	Discharges (3 years)	Nursing index	Nurse Magnet hospital	Technology (of 5)	Patient/ community services (of 8)	NCI cancer center	Hospice/ palliative care
1	Memorial Sloan-Kettering Cancer Center, New York	100.0	69.6	0.77	6,744	1.5	No	5.0	8	Yes	H, P
2	University of Texas M. D. Anderson Cancer Center, Houston	99.1	69.7	0.82	6,967	2.0	Yes	5.0	5	Yes	P
3	Johns Hopkins Hospital, Baltimore	69.0	35.7	0.53	2,423	2.3	Yes	5.0	8	Yes	H, P
4	Mayo Clinic, Rochester, Minn.	60.7	28.2	0.55	5,247	2.8	Yes	4.0	8	Yes	H, P
5	Dana-Farber Cancer Institute, Boston	59.7	35.8	0.64	326	0.8	Yes	2.5	5	Yes	H, P
6	University of Washington Medical Center, Seattle	44.1	14.9	0.60	1,130	2.2	Yes	5.0	7	Yes	H, P
7	Duke University Medical Center, Durham, N.C.	36.8	7.8	0.64	3,305	1.8	No	5.0	8	Yes	H, P
8	University of Chicago Hospitals	36.5	6.9	0.52	1,872	2.3	No	5.0	7	Yes	H, P
9	UCLA Medical Center, Los Angeles	36.5	8.8	0.62	1,651	2.2	Yes	5.0	5	Yes	P
10	University of California, San Francisco Medical Center	36.1	11.8	0.86	1,488	2.3	No	5.0	8	Yes	P
11	H. Lee Moffitt Cancer Center and Research Institute, Tampa	35.6	5.7	0.43	2,145	1.4	No	5.0	8	Yes	H, P
12	University of Pittsburgh Medical Center	35.2	5.9	0.59	2,391	1.9	No	5.0	8	Yes	H, P
13	Cleveland Clinic	34.9	6.8	0.75	3,545	1.5	Yes	5.0	8	Yes	H, P
14	Stanford Hospital and Clinics, Stanford, Calif.	33.9	11.8	0.73	1,225	1.6	No	5.0	7	No	P
15	Massachusetts General Hospital, Boston	33.8	9.5	1.01	2,618	1.9	Yes	5.0	8	Yes	H, P
16	Fox Chase Cancer Center, Philadelphia	33.6	7.2	0.69	1,099	1.6	Yes	4.5	7	Yes	H, P
17	Barnes-Jewish Hospital/Washington University, St. Louis	33.0	3.2	0.64	3,950	1.7	Yes	5.0	8	Yes	H, P
18	University of Michigan Hospitals and Health System, Ann Arbor	32.7	4.5	0.61	2,077	2.4	No	5.0	8	Yes	P
19	Hospital of the University of Pennsylvania, Philadelphia	30.6	7.6	0.96	1,747	1.7	No	5.0	8	Yes	H, P
20	Vanderbilt University Medical Center, Nashville	30.2	4.6	0.75	1,580	1.7	No	5.0	7	Yes	H, P
21	Ohio State University James Cancer Hospital, Columbus	29.9	3.5	0.80	2,885	1.9	No	5.0	8	Yes	H, P
22	University Medical Center, Tucson, Ariz.	29.9	0.9	0.48	664	2.1	Yes	4.5	8	Yes	H, P
23	University of Alabama Hospital at Birmingham	29.7	2.3	0.65	2,022	2.0	Yes	3.5	6	Yes	H, P
24	New York-Presbyterian Univ. Hosp. of Columbia and Cornell	29.3	5.4	0.88	4,349	1.4	No	4.0	8	Yes	H, P
25	University Hospitals of Cleveland	28.9	1.0	0.52	1,447	1.4	No	5.0	8	Yes	H, P
26	Yale-New Haven Hospital, New Haven, Conn.	28.8	0.5	0.55	1,572	2.5	No	4.0	8	Yes	H, P
27	Brigham and Women's Hospital, Boston	28.3	1.3	0.74	1,990	2.3	No	5.0	8	Yes	H, P
28	University of Wisconsin Hospital and Clinics, Madison	28.2	1.6	0.40	1,316	1.7	No	4.0	7	Yes	
29	University of Minnesota Medical Center, Minneapolis	28.1	1.0	0.63	1,391	1.8	No	5.0	8	Yes	H, P
30	University of Virginia Medical Center, Charlottesville	27.5	0.9	0.74	1,791	2.0	No	5.0	8	Yes	H, P
31	University of California, Irvine Medical Center, Orange	27.5	0.3	0.54	545	1.7	Yes	4.0	8	Yes	H, P
32	University of Colorado Hospital, Denver	27.3	1.9	0.64	646	2.1	Yes	4.0	7	Yes	P
33	University of California, San Diego Medical Center	27.0	0.0	0.44	642	1.9	No	4.0	7	Yes	H, P
34	University of Utah Hospitals and Clinics, Salt Lake City	26.7	0.3	0.61	967	2.2	No	5.0	8	Yes	P
35	Rush University Medical Center, Chicago	26.1	0.3	0.65	1,298	2.0	Yes	5.0	8	No	H, P
36	William Beaumont Hospital, Royal Oak, Mich.	26.0	0.6	0.70	2,972	1.8	Yes	4.0	8	No	H, P
37	Northwest Community Hospital, Arlington Heights, Ill.	25.7	0.0	0.51	1,316	2.0	Yes	4.0	6	No	H, P
38	Lehigh Valley Hospital, Allentown, Pa.	25.7	0.0	0.62	1,509	2.0	Yes	4.0	8	No	H, P
39	Henry Ford Hospital, Detroit	25.6	1.6	0.70	1,540	1.7	No	5.0	8	No	H, P
40	University of North Carolina Hospitals, Chapel Hill	25.5	0.9	0.83	1,492	1.9	No	5.0	8	Yes	H, P
41	Oregon Health and Science University Hospital, Portland	25.3	0.9	0.79	788	2.1	No	5.0	8	Yes	H, P
42	Beth Israel Deaconess Medical Center, Boston	25.3	0.8	0.61	1,555	1.6	No	5.0	7	No	H, P
43	Dartmouth-Hitchcock Medical Center, Lebanon, N.H.	25.3	0.0	0.79	1,165	1.6	Yes	5.0	8	Yes	H, P
44	Evanston Northwestern Healthcare, Evanston, Ill.	25.1	0.6	0.61	1,795	1.2	No	5.0	8	No	H, P
45	Riverside Methodist Hospital-Ohio Health, Columbus	25.0	0.0	0.60	1,549	1.4	Yes	4.0	8	No	H, P
46	University Hospital, Albuquerque, N.M.	24.8	0.3	0.67	381	2.0	No	4.0	8	Yes	H, P
47	Harper University Hospital, Detroit	24.8	0.3	0.71	1,935	0.9	No	4.5	7	Yes	H, P
48	Thomas Jefferson University Hospital, Philadelphia	24.6	0.4	0.86	1,787	1.7	No	5.0	8	Yes	H, P
49	Greater Baltimore Medical Center	24.6	0.0	0.47	1,361	1.2	No	4.0	8	No	H, P
50	Sarasota Memorial Hospital, Fla.	24.6	0.0	0.58	1,728	1.6	Yes	3.0	7	No	H, P

Note: Apparent ties are due to rounding. Terms are explained on Page 110.

More information at www.usnews.com/besthospitals

6. Information on Cancer Treatment Centers

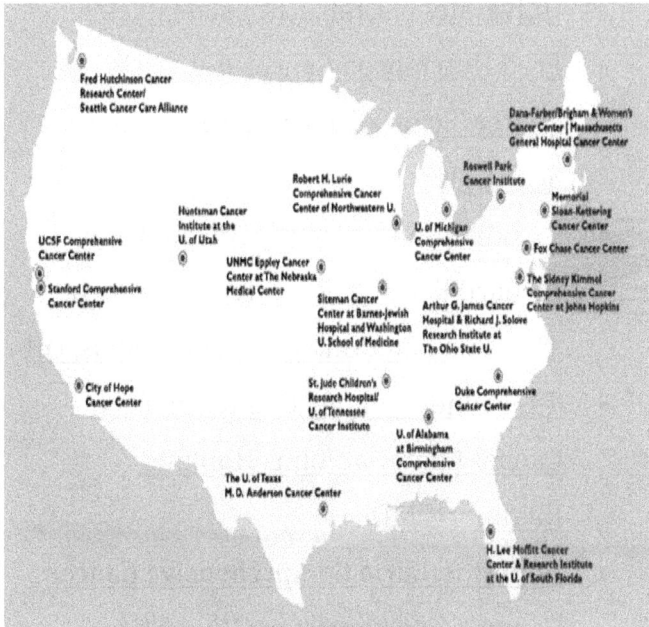

The NCCN Member Institutions are:

- City of Hope Cancer Center, Los Angeles, CA

- Dana-Farber/Brigham & Women's Cancer Center | Massachusetts General Hospital Cancer Center, Boston, MA

- Duke Comprehensive Cancer Center, Durham, NC

- Fox Chase Cancer Center, Philadelphia, PA

112

- Huntsman Cancer Institute at the University of Utah, Salt Lake City, UT
- Fred Hutchinson Cancer Research Center/Seattle Cancer Care Alliance, Seattle, WA
- Arthur G. James Cancer Hospital and Richard J. Solove Research Institute at The Ohio State University, Columbus, OH
- The Sidney Kimmel Comprehensive Cancer Center at Johns Hopkins, Baltimore, MD
- Robert H. Lurie Comprehensive Cancer Center of Northwestern University, Chicago, IL
- Memorial Sloan-Kettering Cancer Center, New York, NY
- H. Lee Moffitt Cancer Center & Research Institute at the University of South Florida, Tampa, FL
- Roswell Park Cancer Institute, Buffalo, NY
- Siteman Cancer Center at Barnes-Jewish Hospital and Washington University School of Medicine, St. Louis, MO

- St. Jude Children's Research Hospital/University of Tennessee Cancer Institute, Memphis, TN
- Stanford Comprehensive Cancer Center, Stanford, CA
- University of Alabama at Birmingham Comprehensive Cancer Center, Birmingham, AL
- UCSF Comprehensive Cancer Center, San Francisco, CA
- University of Michigan Comprehensive Cancer Center, Ann Arbor, MI
- UNMC Eppley Cancer Center at The Nebraska Medical Center, Omaha, NE
- The University of Texas M. D. Anderson Cancer Center, Houston, TX.

ELIZABETH

A Portrait

Elizabeth at Age 28

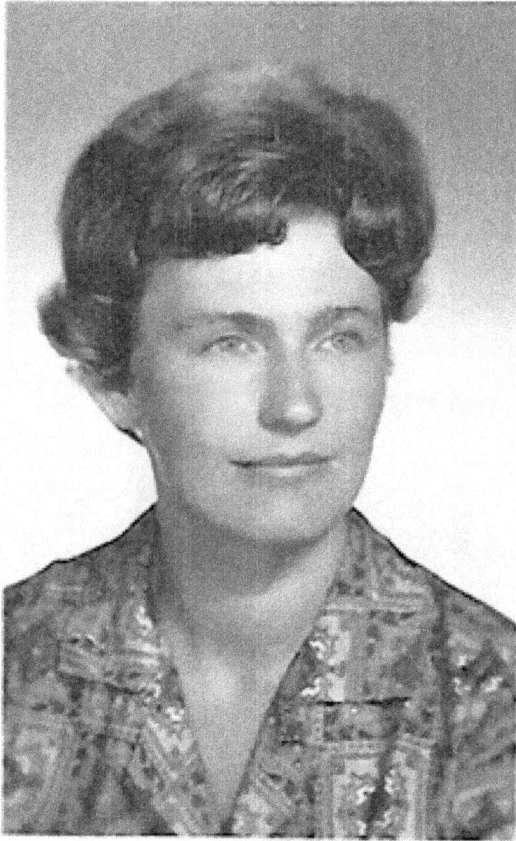

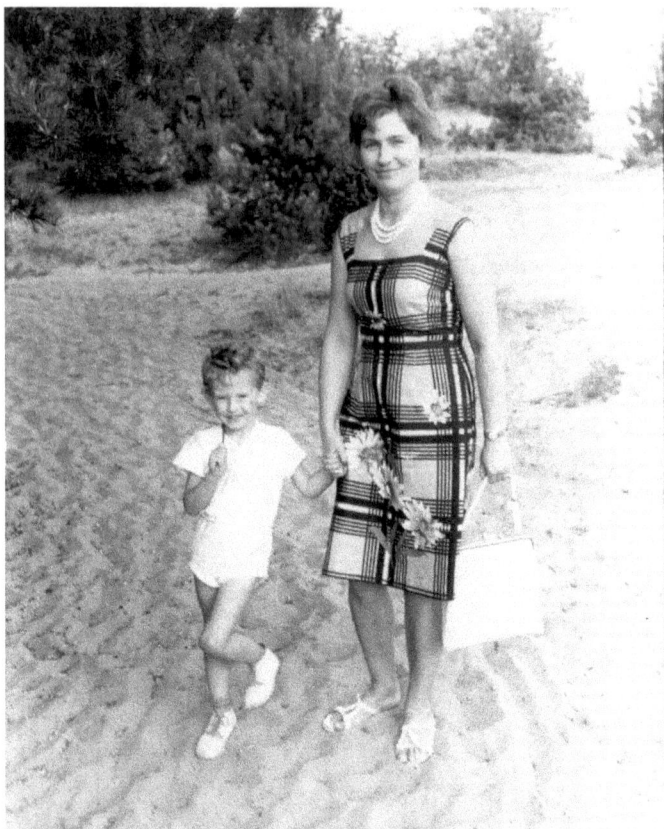

Elizabeth at Age 29

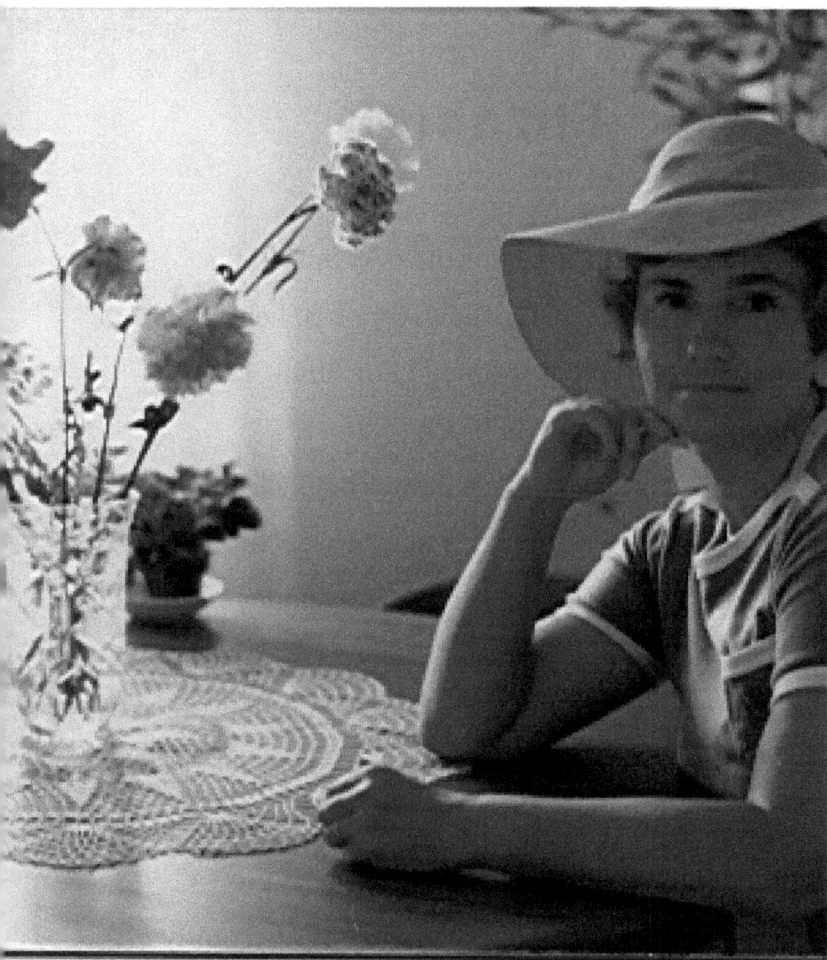

Elizabeth at Age 57

Elizabeth

I saw Elizabeth for the first time in the company canteen. Somehow, I spotted her in the large crowd milling around at lunchtime. I asked Joe,

"Do you know that lady, who is she?"

"Forget that lady, she is married; besides, she is inaccessible. She is constantly under siege by a bunch in our office and from elsewhere. I have not heard of any successes. I am friends with her and do a little flirting, but that is where my dreams end."

I tried not to think of "that lady" too much. Nevertheless my troubled mind constantly veered towards Elizabeth at a time when my own marriage to Cynthia was nothing but trouble. It was difficult to verbalize what Elizabeth's attraction was. She certainly was pretty in all aspects, but not in the way of a stereotypical beauty. There was this something in her that drove the guys to extraordinary efforts to get at least a smile or a shred of attention. Just to be in her presence gave these guys a high. The intensity of that pull became conspicuously apparent some time later. Occasionally, I visited the neighboring department where she worked, for purely business reasons. I never spoke to her and was never introduced. Nevertheless, these trips became something more than business, just seeing her in passing was a good, soothing experience for the day. I learned much later that she had asked Joe,

"Do you know that guy who is visiting here from Department X, can you tell me something about him?"

Nothing happened for a while except that it came to the point where my thinking about Elizabeth became obsessive. Then, one day, there was an announcement that Department Y was being dissolved and its staff would be dispersed among the other offices. Elizabeth ended up in my department working for me! The days became one uninterrupted string of roller coaster rides. Spiritual highs at work after devastating and excruciatingly hard times at home with Cynthia. I could be around Elizabeth for eight hours! Talk to her at will! Soon Elizabeth filled my days completely and I was slowly but steadily becoming more involved with her.

Nevertheless, I had to maintain the role of the boss with consummate propriety required by my position and by my own boss, who was a stickler for discipline and propriety. Also, having a lot of mental baggage from the past, I did not allow myself to dream of her having anything more to do with me than a routine work relationship. The problem that very soon surfaced was the constant stream of men from within the department wanting to have a word with Elizabeth, which made working at her job difficult. My boss noticed that and did not wait long to summon me into his office.

"Mister So, what will we do with Elizabeth?"

"Sir, leave it to me, I will come up with something."

"Very well then, that is all I wanted from you for the moment."

That was his style. His words were like a military dismissal. I turned around and left not knowing what in the world I would do. I came up with a scheme by which I designated half an hour in the morning and half in the afternoon when it was permitted to talk to Elizabeth on non-business matters. This was posted at her workstation and strictly enforced.

In the meantime, my marriage to Cynthia entered the final phase of falling apart. I had invested so many emotions in her and my devotion was so complete, that the end of that marriage and my absolute helplessness was crushing me, my budding feelings for Elizabeth notwithstanding. One day Elizabeth asked to speak to me privately.

"Sven, I need a divorce, do you know a lawyer I could trust and turn to?"

I did not waste a minute. To my surprise and happiness, Elizabeth accepted my shy advances and we eventually became lovers, while both our marriages were dissolving and heading for divorce. She had a much harder time because of her son, Jack, who was one year old. Since we both had to uphold appearances for a while and could not use our respective homes, we met and made love under circumstances unimaginable for a western person not living under communism. In short, it was impossible to get a hotel room, because anybody wanting one had to show a reason and this could only be official business. Thus, we met in all kinds of places that make me shudder even today. I was sick with worry. I worried that this was not conducive to Elizabeth's receiving gratification and that it was degrading. I tried my utmost to bring her to orgasm, but having never had one did not even know what one was. This became my obsession and I totally disregarded my own pleasures, deciding that our lovemaking would never mean anything to me without Elizabeth being gratified. On one of our lucky days we got the apartment of a friend who was on vacation. We made love and suddenly Elizabeth started behaving unusually. Her breathing became heavy and fast, soon she broke out into a spasmodic sobbing. Frightened, I asked, "Elizabeth, what is the matter, have I done something wrong, did I hurt you?"

She wrapped her arms tightly around me, put her lips close to my ear, and whispered, "It happened, it happened!"

I could not think of anything to say, I clutched to her so close that I thought I would push her inside me. The bliss that came over me was so intense that I thought my chest would burst. Only later did I start reflecting. She had five years of marriage to this guy who was considered vastly superior to me as a male specimen. Later when we openly got together and married, people shook their heads in wonderment. "What has gotten into that woman?" Even some of my so-called friends were at a loss to understand her choice. This is how our journey together began. Having concluded with absolute conviction that I am not lovable to women, I could never get rid of my own bewilderment at what has happened. One time I could not hold back the temptation and asked.

"Elizabeth, why did you marry me?"

"Oh... because there was no mother-in-law involved."

It was true that in her previous marriage she had suffered greatly from her then mother-in- law. Obviously, I was at a loss to know whether this was just a flippant answer or what. Unfortunately, the too short thirty-six years of our marriage was marked by answers like this whenever I tried to draw out and make her verbalize some inner feelings. On the other hand, she was always very specific when it came to expressing anger with me over what she perceived as my failings.

From that moment, our intimacy became stronger. I relaxed and became confident and my previous troubles sustaining an erection were gone. I made sure that Elizabeth was gratified and my own gratification was secondary. Elizabeth moved in with me and we became a functioning family. Elizabeth was moving along toward enjoying sex and any inhibitions between us vanished; we could talk, experiment, and to my immeasurable happiness she displayed a basic, but restrained, sexuality. This became, while not the only the only bond between us, a strong foundation for years to come and to the very end, even during her illness. Some of the most memorable moments and there were many, were our vacations at the Baltic seashore. There, we found a miles-long desolate beach with nobody around. Jack was put down for naps sleep in the afternoons and we made love between sand dunes or sometimes in the bushes nearby. This is when I discovered what I should have considered a delightful "kink" in her nature. I was always deliberately building shelters and obstructions, so nobody could see us even from the border guard watchtower miles away. Elizabeth always looked at my efforts with amusement and was totally unconcerned about somebody seeing us. One time we were in the bushes and a man happened to walk by. I immediately got shy, but Elizabeth pulled me down and we proceeded. I was flustered, but Elizabeth was quite amused and happy with the incident—Nicos's teachings vindicated. There were slight disappointments on my part, because it seemed that I never had enough. We settled into a routine where subtle signals passed between us with me never daring to push my way; I would never contemplate it anyway, because I was unable to perform under the slightest notion of not being wanted. There is another image from that period that I hold in my memory, and it has not faded in the least; Elizabeth in a light body-shaped dress with flowery patterns, slender and so happy, the sea and the white bright sand in the background.

Soon, I realized how rare our situation was. In all the marriages I saw around me, including that of my mentor Nicos, sex and related matters were excruciatingly difficult issues and most of the time spoilers of marriage. Often the husband would roam around in search for fulfillment, mostly in vain. My social surroundings became a kaleidoscopic pattern of cheatings, breakups and bizarre, juicy social events. That meant that Elizabeth was constantly under "attack" and since "all is fair in love and war," I would have to be on guard from even my friends. Looking back at those times, it was

127

remarkable how intense and how much mental preoccupation and energy my friends and acquaintances put into the pursuit of the elusive goal of finding a fulfilling sex partner.

Despite Elizabeth's very strong attractiveness, which meant that she had to deal with advances from men at work and sometimes from total strangers, throughout her daily activities calm and confidence came finally my way. I was not racked by bouts of jealousy anymore; seeing her enjoyment with our being together, learning more about her views and feelings about men and human relations, convinced me that she was very comfortable and urges to seek excitement outside our relationship did not enter her mind. If they did, she would chase them out. She was basically a much disciplined lady. She raised that question herself once:

"Sven, I wonder if you sometimes have doubts about me being faithful. You must think of the fact that I cheated with you on Wieslaw?"

"Elizabeth, it may be difficult for you to believe this, but that thought has not even entered my mind. Your marriage was a mistake and so was mine. They were falling apart badly; we should think that they never existed. I would not call it cheating and I never ever will doubt you."

We never talked about this subject again. What gave me greater reassurances of my correct perception, although it was coupled with some hurt, was an incident that took place years later. We were by then in the USA, Elizabeth got very upset with me about something, and in anger she said,

"In Italy"—she had been in Rome alone for some time—"those gorgeous Italians were after me constantly, I was absolutely faithful to you even in thought, should I be regretting it now?"

After I finished writing this narrative, Mary— she was with Elizabeth in Rome the whole time for the same reasons—emigrated, called me and mentioned that she has just seen Kubrick's film the "Eyes Wide Shut." I said, "I consider the subject he has raised very important. Men and some women struggle mightily with these problems, which seem to come to us from the depth of primordial times."

"Yes, I agree, I saw here in New York a man, probably Italian, in the subway train. He was so handsome; I could not let my eyes off him. I cannot forget him and it was such a long time ago."

She called back after a short while and said, "I have to tell you something and I hope you will not be upset about it now. In Rome, Elizabeth had to deal with these Italians all the time. One time there was a bus driver so irresistibly handsome and he would not quit coming on to Elizabeth. She finally agreed for him to see her the next day. She asked me to be with her at all times and we spent, the three of us, most of that day with him driving us around Rome and sightseeing. The whole thing ended at that."

And so, that story had made a full circle, after thirty-one years.

There were other instances, which faded from view, but a couple of scenes I kept and have cherished in my memory very vividly, never to forget. Shortly after we established our household in that one-room apartment where the two-year old Jack was sleeping in a corner crib, I came out from under the shower and there was Elizabeth, naked. Her exquisitely shaped slender body stretched out on the floor on the carpet – our rickety bed was noisy and we always were careful not wake the child. In the dim light of the small lamp I saw her face glowing with such intensity and anticipation that I froze for a moment, taken by surprise. She stretched her arms out to me. We did not go to bed for a long time, we just lay there naked on the floor in a tight embrace. Elizabeth never verbalized her feelings toward me although she was such an outspoken lady, if she disliked something she came right out with it and with precision. A declaration of love I heard one or two times only, much, much later. Was she too proud? Most of the time, I had to guess her attachment to me from her behavior.

A second reassuring but excruciatingly painful scene took place when I left Poland and she had to stay behind because of custody issues over Jack. It was the final goodbye, half way to the border. Elizabeth broke into such despair and crying that my friend Jacob had to support her and help her into the car. Through uncontrolled sobbing she repeatedly said, "I will never see you again!"

Elizabeth was always very restrained in expressing her emotions, except for those of anger. For three long months I waited for her in Rome, and that scene more than anything put me into an indescribable state of mental anguish and pain; to think now of all the bitter suffering we had to go through, why?

This brings me to one other aspect of Elizabeth's make-up. Polish society was and is permeated by anti-Semitism. It is so engrained in the common man that it caused Begin to state, "They suck it out with their mother's milk."

Communism suppressed the manifestation of that, but later used it for its own political ends. From the time they took power and long after the war it could not erase that aspect from the minds of the common man and probably did not want to, it was an old historical and cherished characteristic of the Poles.

Elizabeth came from a lower-class factory-hand family where anti-Semitism was strong and almost a spiritual element second only to religion. The jokes, outrageous stories and most exciting gossip were about Jews, although very few were left in Poland after the holocaust. Some survivors, barely alive, were murdered by mob action in the infamous purely anti-Jewish riots in the town of Kielce. In juxtaposition to this was the amazing fact that one could find Poles in different strata of that society completely devoid of any traces of anti-Semitism and ashamed and chagrinned by this national situation. Those were the people that made my life and progress in that society possible, for a while at least, until the government and the Communist Party unleashed the pent up national anti-Semitism. Although to protect me, some of my Polish coworkers and friends from college made an effort that was heroic and dangerous for them, this was the last straw that forced me out of Poland and brought us to the parting scene described above. It is remarkable that women had this anti-Semitic trait much less often than men and often married Jews, which led to their ostracism by their own social peers. Obviously, Elizabeth was such a woman, absolutely devoid of any prejudice, strong and independent in the face of her family's display of disapproval. The subject of Jews often came up in her family settings—Mother and brothers and the entire milieu of relatives. Elizabeth mocked them mercilessly and her tongue was sharper than a razor blade. It is worth mentioning that when Elizabeth went to visit her parents for an hour or so, I was waiting in the car around the corner. She became an American citizen with great pride, and after repeated visits to Poland to see her mother she said after one of her returns,

"When my Mother dies, I will never set foot in Poland again!"

This in itself was such an immense departure from the typical "patriotic" Polish attitude, which implies that there is something unique and holy mysterious to be a Pole, that it amazed me and gratified me immensely, because I felt exactly the same—to never set foot in Poland again, although I have left magnificent friends behind and that is one very sad aspect of it all. From the perspective of time and since meeting Vicky it seems even more amazing. Vicky is a highly educated PhD; she seemed to be one of those Polish women with no traces of anti-Semitism and was seemingly fond of my company. Nevertheless she used the phrase "I am a pure Pole," that is, as opposed to an impure Pole like—maybe me. Lech Walesa had used the same phrase when running for president of Poland against his opponent, whose great–grandparents had some traces of Jewish blood in their lineage. This was to reassure the populace that not a drop of Jewish blood would rule over them.

America was incredibly good to us. We came with literally nothing, but in a short time built together and attained the living status and quality of life of the upper middle class. I spoke English, but Elizabeth got a job without a word of English. Even though it was technical work, still the people who hired her were extraordinary. We shortly started looking at houses — Elizabeth's dream was to have one of her own—

but the idea it seemed so remote. She mentioned some of our escapades at her office and shortly after that the president summoned her to his office. She was sure it was to let her go. The president said,

"Elizabeth, I heard from Melanie"— his secretary—"that you are contemplating buying a house, I have spoken to my friend who is a bank manager, and the company has vouched for you, go get a loan for as much as you need."

We lived the American dream, and after years of hard work we built a gorgeous retirement house to Elizabeth's specifications and were prepared to live a few tranquil years after a life full of turbulence, danger, worry and hard work. We were hoping to savor our undiminished and enduring love. Disaster struck just at the very threshold of our retirement; Elizabeth died at the age of sixty-two. The light of the days went out for me permanently. It looks like some abjectly cruel joker selected that very moment to strike, or is it all blind chance? The Franciscan friar, father Juniper tackled that very question as early or late—depending on one's view as the year 1714. He wanted to find out if we all live and die by chance, or are creatures "under God's control." He worked under the assumption that God is just and fair because that is what he wanted to prove. After finishing his investigation and presenting his results, the church authorities ordered him to be burned at the stake with all his works, so we do not know what he found out, or can we guess? Nevertheless, I am thinking of presenting our story to the believers in Divine Justice, for their collection of supportive facts. I am sure that their answer would be, "Unknown to us is the wisdom of God." But then, why should I expose myself to a mockingly offensive answer of an ignorant kind? It is injurious to a rational mind.

A Short Summation

Now, whoever stops me and cares to ask what kind of woman Elizabeth was, I have a short summation that I am placing below.

That question always starts me on a difficult search for words and what I usually come up with seems so inadequate and clumsy. What follows below is an attempt at an answer without the pressure of the moment and overriding my verbal awkwardness.

The short phrase I use if I want to avoid saying much more is, "She was an unusual and atypical woman." I then follow with a succinct comparison understandable to most that sounds like this, "She was a Rolls Royce Silver Cloud limited edition of a woman." It mostly stops there, but if pressed for details I go on.

The crucial and rare quality of the woman was that she had some sex drive and was interested in and enjoyed sex as a very important part of our lives, undiminished to the last. That alone most often predicates the course of a marriage. She was disciplined about it, but none too sparing and there were no signs of her seeking thrills on the outside. In general, ours was what I would call a high intensity body contact relationship; we were fond of each other's bodies. Uniquely, she lacked or had very weak pheromone receptors; therefore she did not react as many women do by wetting her pants at the sight of a soap opera male. I therefore was quite confident that she would not run off with a Tom Selleck type or fantasize about some idol during our intimate moments. She recognized male handsomeness in a somewhat detached way. She would not go for the knockout guys, courted or not. She had her own set of criteria very much apart from that of much of the female crowd and in that I found my fortunate chances. A telling and gratifying example was her attitude toward the Clinton phenomenon, where almost universally women got dreamily infatuated with that character. Elizabeth considered him a repulsive boar of a man.

Complementing this was her powerful attractiveness and the pull she exerted on men. That was sometimes a source of irritation and it needed maneuvering to stay clear of involvements, at the same time keeping civil and not meting out hurt. She was very good at that, polite, friendly and calm unless someone crossed the barrier, then she would be mercilessly violent. Whenever a woman in social settings complained about not being able to deflect somebody's advances I would say, "Ask that guy to harass Elizabeth, he may not live after that and your problem will be solved."

Her popularity was also a source of pride for her and for me. Most of the time, she managed things smoothly and that gave us material for discussions and wonderment about human nature. One light moment stands out in my memory. I had an employee by the name of Peter, Pretty Peter they called him. A poor performer, he spent most of his time at women's workstations. He gravitated heavily toward Elizabeth. Any time I turned away, he was there at Elizabeth's side. I was more concerned about what my Big Boss, who had an eagle eye and was fierce and dictatorial, was going to say, rather than about Peter charming Elizabeth; her reaction was:

"I have to admit, he is dashingly handsome, it is fun to watch how these women here are all getting giddy over Peter and casting an evil eye on me.

One day the big boss called me into his office and said,

"Mister So, our work load is falling off and we have an opportunity to get rid of some non-performers. I have selected two guys from your department, make preparations."

One of the guys he selected was Pretty Peter. After that incident the kidding never stopped.

"Remember when you fired Peter, you must have been really jealous..."

On occasion the situation turned very uncomfortable, like the time she had to leave her job because her boss (she went to another company after we got involved) fell hopelessly in love and confessed to Elizabeth that he could not go on. His marriage was suffering and he was unable to work with her presence in the office, with no hope of "getting her for life." This was a reaction she often encountered, serious passions "for life", the "only woman" et cetera. I could well understand the man's mental condition; I was in exactly the same situation before we married, although I do not know if I could have contained myself being around her every day at work without hope. Probably I could have, but with great suffering, therefore I made no comments about her boss's behavior, but felt terrible because of the trouble she had to go through.

She was very pretty, not flashily beautiful in the proverbial way, although I often heard "beautiful," and I took it as applying to her as a whole rather than to her purely facial attributes. She was calmly self-confident without a trace of the flirtatious or coquettish. She had to deal with a lot of advances without using that. Amazingly, she was always ready with witty, pleasing answers. On the other hand, when something displeased her, she was always ready with sharp slashing responses. Men as well as women liked to talk to her and simply be in her company. Men usually are intimidated by what commonly is considered a beauty. They seem to view those flashy women as capricious, demanding, unstable and not for everyday life. A fling, yes, but no serious involvement. When a woman like Elizabeth comes along they seem to think, "This is it, a dream come true, I cannot live without her." She often faced that situation as a young woman and less often, but still occasionally, after she married. For me it definitely was a "dream come true" and I often rubbed my eyes in disbelief.

It is universal knowledge that the true nature of marriage comes out only after the wedding and the situation usually drifts into hell sooner or later. I vividly remember a visit from my school friend Ed Buttermilk. I had not seen him for a few years and greeted him with open arms and a loud, cheerful "My goodness, Buttermilk, how are you!"

"Do not call me Buttermilk, I got married and took my wife's name. My name now is Nakedman." (a somewhat imprecise translation from the Polish, but expressing the idea)

"All right, how is your marriage going?"

"Just typical, there are only three problems—sex, money matters and dealing with children."

Money matters: Elizabeth was a superbly elegant dresser. That usually implies huge and wasteful expense. The way she handled that was always within the bounds of our budget, besides, she worked and contributed. That area turned into pure joy where I often had to urge her to buy something to dramatically complement her prettiness. I could always expect what became a constant refrain in social gatherings. "Elizabeth is smashingly elegant tonight!" Dressing Elizabeth was definitely a matter to pay attention to with considerable gratification. Still, in Poland she came home one day and said,

"I got transferred to this other division and I cannot find out why, it is not a worse position but the lack of explanation bothers me."

As we found out later through the grapevine, the president's wife demanded that Elizabeth be out of sight because she could not stand her being so much better dressed than she was, when she, the top man's wife, showed up. This happened when I came back from the Far East and brought a number of exotic outfits, which, amazingly, were to Elizabeth's taste.

Although women in her workplaces gravitated to her and sought her company she often felt petty jealousies and unpleasant motives like idle curiosity and hunting for a chink in her seemingly perfect bearing and allure. Therefore, she had a cautious and ambivalent attitude toward women. I only now realize the blessing of it when I encounter the contemporary and the older man-hating feminists. Elizabeth was totally devoid of this. Not one time did I hear a stereotypical remark about men. She had a select circle of female friends. The information and gossip she brought back from these contacts showed over and over again how different her perceptions and reactions were from what was found in that collection of females. The short info sessions after her return from women- only encounters left me always in an elated state, realizing how fortunate I was to have Elizabeth. Some of the ladies had a designated day, monthly or fortnightly, when they succumbed to the awful urges of their husbands. That was somewhat verifiable information from slips in my conversations with the guys.

She was very comfortable in male surroundings, which was mostly what she had all her working years. Her ever-ready combativeness kept any bothersome transgressions in check and that always set the stage for **relatively** smooth "sailing." I, on the other hand, was always trying to avoid confrontations, and definitely tried not to give her any excuse for one. Elizabeth did not seek or provoke confrontations, but when it looked like there was one in the offing; she utterly enjoyed destroying her opponent without mercy or remorse. In Springfield, after Elizabeth had become quite proficient in English, I came home one day to see her dressed and made up smashingly.

"Elizabeth, what is this, where are you going?"

"I have an appointment with the bank manager; I am going to give him a bloody nose like he has never had before—how do I look?"

Her eyes flashed with mischievous excitement.

"Well, if I were him, I would lose my ability to speak."

The next day I was in the bank for something.

"Hi, Mr. Sonnenberg, your wife was here yesterday. We had quite a lot of fun. We have never seen our manager in such a nervous hurry."

The feminist movement dismayed her. She felt that it hurt her at work by creating a tense and fearful atmosphere full of hidden and fuzzy dealings and scheming. She hated that and was unable to scheme herself and always preferred a frontal attack. The feminists did not help her in getting responsibilities, promotions, et cetera. When approached to join any of those female organizations at work she always refused. She felt that the movement took away her traditional feminine advantages in dealing with issues. The perverse situation brought about by the militant feminist movement was very obvious in the big Rochester Corporation where we worked together for a while. Women were advanced for show, for obscure political reasons that had nothing to do with genuine work performance.

A married woman becomes emotionally restless very soon. The adolescent dreams of Prince Charming on a White Horse never fade. The realization soon sets in that it is much worse than just not having gotten the Prince. Demands and dissatisfactions start, the bashing becomes relentless, "You could get a better job and the Johnston's have this and that." "Why are we living in this God-forsaken place?" If the woman is asexual, which is mostly the case, or the husband is unable to strike any spark in her, that then sets the stage for a grim and resentful coexistence until the blow-up. Even in a reasonably satisfying marriage, the Prince Charming dreams never fade. They leave unspecified longings that erupt now and then in outbursts that seem totally irrational to the husband and impossible to understand; emotional volatility becomes a curse. * See footnote

I will always remember a fragment from an article depicting a short scene,
The husband: "But Honey, this is what you wanted!"

"Yes, that is what I wanted five minutes ago."

Elizabeth had very faint traces of that, if any, and I often wondered if she had the Prince Charming syndrome hidden away deep down. It appeared that she was blessedly devoid of that typical female attribute as well, but it is difficult for me to be absolutely certain. She never displayed any dreamy longings for a glamorous dance party somewhere, a voyage to an exotic place or a meeting with so and so, et cetera et cetera. She was focused on family and very disciplined about it, very practical without a fault. She expected the same from me and would not have tolerated my going with buddies for drinking or cards or hunting. Luckily, I was not much interested in this typical male behavior.

My family and Elizabeth was my focus; she came along to the shooting range. We spent no time away from each other except for work. The one frequent grudge she had was my dedication to work, which was a necessity for us new immigrants. She was superbly logical in her views and opinions. I do not remember a hostile confrontation about political or social issues. We seemed to be able to rationally explore differences and come to a compromise. In spite of her uncommon logic, she was sometimes very unfair and hurtful in her remarks; spitefulness was often the mark of her responses. She was utterly unable to apologize for the deep slashing verbal hurts she meted out sometimes even when she realized that she was wrong. Her anger was always close to the surface. Any displeasure or seeming provocation brought out a strong reaction. After one of those I said, "Elizabeth, all these years I have never heard an apology for the nasty things you sometimes come up with."

"I am too perfect to apologize for anything."

"Granted, nearly perfect you are, but in the department of bridling your anger you are sometimes lacking."

"You have an uncommon wife; besides, a husband is also for venting one's frustrations upon."

She was well aware of her superior uniqueness and to argue against that I could not. There was though something deep in her psyche, perhaps from her childhood when she witnessed her mother's very unhappy marriage full of recriminations and animosity. I once said,

"Elizabeth, considering everything, how can you ever get angry with me?"

"I do not know, usually I cannot help it."

Late in her illness she started a diary, which I read after her death. In it, she talks about her first days in Carolina before she got ill, also, about her settling in her dream house, built and arranged exactly as she wished, no expenses barred. She wrote about her night dreams and emotions and how she easily got a satisfying job. One of her lines reads: "I felt that I was on top of the world." She never let me know about that feeling. On the contrary, she became moody and often unfair, complaining about trifles in my behavior. Was it the unrecognized signs of the developing illness? I wondered often at the time, did she really love me. The dialog from the Fiddler on the Roof comes to mind.

Tevye asks his wife, "Do you love me?"

"I have raised your children, I have cooked for you, and I have washed your clothes."

"Yes, yes, I know, but do you love me?"

Tevye cannot get a straight answer.

In all our more than thirty-six years together, I remember one specific time when Elizabeth clearly said, that she loved me. It was late in our marriage, so sudden and out of context, that it etched itself into memory. Sitting close on the couch and turning suddenly to me, without anything to prompt her, she said,

"I love you so much."

I hugged her and kissed her in response, but did not say anything. I do not know how I could so stupidly forget the basic tenet that for women sweet words sometimes mean more than deeds; that omission will haunt me forever. That was one time she said it in such a spontaneous and emotional way and I would surely remember if there were others. I was simply assuming that she did love me from her behavior and actions and her dedication. Very often, in the evening when we went to bed and got into a tight embrace she would sigh a deep sigh of relaxation and relief, and say "We have to go through all the tribulations of a day for this moment." During days whenever she was tired and needed a rest or a nap, she never went on the settee or bed alone. She always would say, "Let's snuggle up for a bit, I need a rest." Needless to say I always eagerly obliged and there we were in the closest possible embrace.

She was a superior mother, very caring, dedicated, but a strict disciplinarian. She kept a perfect balance between her attention to the child and the relationship between us. We always had vacations together as a family. This was a yearly ritual and we traveled all over the U.S. Never, ever was there any tension between us caused by child issues (See Ed Buttermilk).

When she got ill, I went wild with activity trying to save her; only that kept shreds of sanity within me. Although I badgered her about scores of things to do every day, and was insanely frustrated when she was difficult about it, I have to say in retrospect that she was heroic throughout the entire ordeal. My life is shattered now and I do not see any possibility of mending it, even a little bit. Why should I? The memories of Elizabeth's suffering will never leave me; they cloud every day and the so-called joys of life with darkness.

I went to the Wailing Wall in Jerusalem to touch it and to put in a plea to God. I could not concentrate to formulate a wish. I stood there in confusion, my hand on the Wall, unable to say anything. I went away in inner turmoil and walked around and then went back to try again. This is what I put forward,

"God! If you have custody of her, I beg you to make her happy and make her understand how much I loved her."

Strange and inexplicable that I turned to God
after He allowed such a calamity!

Two years have passed since I lost her.

Almost three weeks from now would have been
her 64th birthday.

First day of Summer 2000
North Carolina

A Rather Long Footnote

This footnote might be redundant. Nevertheless,
it is tempting to add some observations to show
how much Elizabeth was different from the
female mainstream.

I met the ladies from her circle of friends
at family or social occasions. It was quite obvious
that when they were frankly expressing their
thoughts they implied to Elizabeth, in an indirect
way that because of her appeal she could have
done so much better than selecting me. Equally
not hurtful to me, but rather amusing, was that
some of my male so-called friends thought

likewise. This was the widespread perception of those ladies of me, "A very nice guy, but..."

How do I know what the ladies thought? Very simple, I listened in on the conversations between the women when they were discussing men or reminiscing about their younger years and suitors they had rejected,

"He was a nice guy, but too short..."

"He had such a strangely unsymmetrical face

"He was already balding..."

Elizabeth listened, but never came forward with a list of her own boyfriends or men she rejected. In conversations between us she sometimes remembered her young years and some of the heart-broken and disappointed boys or young men. This was with a mixture of pride and sadness for their misfortunes. "Frank broke into tears and said he would join the army, and expected to get killed." Once she ran into that very guy after a few years, in the street, in Warsaw. She said, "My heart jumped" and then she added, "I wonder what that was all about?"

An episode she was rather proud of happened during her last year in high school when she was eighteen or nineteen. There was an issue where she was in danger of being punished for something and one of the boys insisted on taking the blame. In the course of deliberating on how to handle the situation, he said, "It is worth dying for Elizabeth."

It was very easy to get into big trouble in those days for the minutest infraction against the communist oppression. In spite of a number of possibilities and sometimes pressure from her mother, who of course had likes and dislikes, I never heard from Elizabeth, "If I had done this or married that guy...", even in anger.

I just came across a Rabbi's confession, which shows a not-so-untypical situation in a "mature" marriage.

"In my previous books, I have always thanked my wife, Debbie, last, in the spirit of saving the best for the summit and conclusion. But any wife who endures a rabbi-husband spending a year writing a book about sex deserves to be thanked first. And although by the book's publication date she will have changed her last name to Smith and had cosmetic surgery so that none of her friends recognize her, I do want to thank my extraordinary wife for all her devotion and support. Of course, there was that time last week when she screamed at the top of her lungs, **"I've had it with you, and I should have listened to my mother. I could have done so much better than you. Johnny, who I dated before you, is now a plumber earning three times your salary. Even your stupid books never sell!"** So Debbie, wherever you are, thanks for leaving some cold meatballs in the freezer. They're still keeping me going."

All kinds of things are said in marital scenes. Elizabeth never came even close to remotely saying something like this, even in a fit of anger. Of course, one never knows what goes on in the absolute privacy of one's thinking. My assumption that her regrets or hindsight as to what might have been were not very strong is based on the fact that Elizabeth was known not to mince words and to come right out with whatever was on her mind at the moment.

Dwelling on regrets about what seem lost opportunities or having made the wrong choice in selecting a mate is such a common and pervasive practice, especially in marriages that have reached some midpoint. It was sometimes embarrassing to witness the whining in public of some of the then already mature ladies from our circle of acquaintances. Their husbands listened to this and tried to make light of it or turn it into impressions of good-natured kidding. One notorious couple was Henry and Natalie; they attended our rather large social gatherings, the so-called "Elizabeth" parties, famous for good food and "interesting" people. I for one did not know what to make of their public bashing of each other, and I thought, "Maybe it is just their style. They are perhaps too comfortable with each other." Not very long after, they got divorced and had a typical adversarial parting.

Lighter bashing of husbands seemed to be a favored pastime of the ladies. Sometimes one was at a loss to know what was good-natured kidding and what was a serious problem. I remember one time a lady let loose on her husband for "not being able to get it up anymore." She was not yet intoxicated. The husband was crumpled up by the fireplace and did not utter a word. Elizabeth never discussed or exposed details of our private life, at least not in my presence. No "good natured" kidding in public!" If she slipped, and only in a very close circle, with one or two friends present, then that would be the only time and she would be able to apologize to me afterwards.

Why not meet someone and settle for less now? Loneliness is very hard for some and might drive me into an undesirable mental state, if I am not already in one. What can I say to this? Even after so much time has elapsed since I lost Elizabeth, it is still revolting to see so many characteristics in the ladies I meet now that were so blessedly absent in Elizabeth's make up.

A Few Parting Words

Looking back now at all the people I have known, friends, people from work and the many acquaintances I have made over the years, I can see a marital landscape littered with burned out remains and broken up debris. The few marriages that endured are convenience unions of people who have stayed together mainly out of inertia and resignation. They are not good. One of my extroverted friends would confess that in the distant past, when he still made love to his wife she would say to him, in the middle of a session, "Let me doze off now, you go ahead and finish." So, there is that crowded field of men living " lives of quiet desperation" – not so quiet though—when I close my eyes and listen carefully I can hear the moaning and groaning of the multitude. Do women suffer too? That is an emphatic yes, but it is not the same—they are different, more cat like, emotionally self-sufficient and much more easily substituting the physically or emotionally departed man with grandchildren or a couple of pets. They do not have that sexual-emotional complex men do and if it is present, it is much more muted. Lack of male companionship for a woman translates more into material decline than anything else and not so often anymore.

It appears; that our situation –Elizabeth's and mine—was somewhat unique in that sea of misery and it seemed worth a short account, at least. Of course everything was not sunny all of the time. Elizabeth was a highly sensitive woman, proud and sometimes intolerant. It is difficult to see clearly my own flaws, but I am sure she could enumerate them readily. Nevertheless, we always ended up in each other's arms after short times of tension. Ugly fights in a classical sense, we have never had. So, I should consider myself lucky or, more appropriately exceedingly lucky to have had the much desired Elizabeth, even more so, because of my male attributes, which were so undeserving. That feeling of luck, which I am told, I should cherish, is marred and greatly cancelled by the final disaster that befell us.

Evidently the script we were writing by living our lives together in that unique way was not well tolerated, He, The Great One upstairs, seems to prefer presiding over mostly protracted lifelong miseries.

What do I have to say to the young, if some would care to listen? Search; do not tolerate a sub-par relationship. Many prefer to endure a bad union rather than risk the unknown again, but that mostly leads to bitterness and nothing left to look back at. Is there any prescription for action or behavior to follow that would assure a successful relationship? In spite of all the books written there is none. What can one do with a woman, who is as cold as a dead fish and does not care to change or seek help, or with a shallow selfish, petty, and capricious dame, or with a volatile, scheming and unreasonable one in love with herself? Nothing can be done. To change a character of any human being, woman or man is the work of Sisyphus. Unfortunately, it is difficult to know what one is dealing with before one commits, everybody seems so skilled in acting and that is true for both, women and men. In today's world to establish a relationship where there is a mutual tolerance of vices with an underlying foundation of dedication and attachment seems almost impossible, even the willingness to tone down or eliminate the idiosyncrasies of one's personality is of no use in this ever changing feminist-movement-dominated society. That movement and television molds the young generation of women into useless for lasting and meaningful relationships.

HOW OTHER MEN HAVE DEALT TWITH THE ORDEAL

Before we delve into some emotional stories, semi-fictional as to names, I must recall two cases, very close and real to me. These were my work companions and the stories are short, very short.

Religious Frank:

When I learned about his young and beautiful wife having been diagnosed with breast cancer, I said, "Frank I found some place in Texas, where I think you could get good help." Frank's answer was "OK, give me the information, but I must tell you I am leaving it to God, God is in control." She was dead in about six months.

Conrad, who had the will to help,

I lost contact with Conrad for a very long time- we went to different companies. Unexpectedly, there was a call from Conrad, "Sven, I heard through the grapevine that you have a supplementary program for your wife, could you please send me what you have." Some weeks passed and I called, "Conrad did you receive my material?" "Yes, I did, but Lucy refused to even read it, and I am unable to convince her to do anything beyond the doctors' orders." Conrad's wife was dead six month later.

When husbands or companions are confronted by the horrifying fact that his woman or wife has terminal cancer, the reactions are immediate and varied.

He may become instantly angry - moving away from her and ultimately seeking the company and comfort of another- often younger and healthier woman. That is precisely what happened to a number of prominent people, among them politicians. And the latter cases are especially sad for us, because these people routinely lecture us how to behave and hold up in front of themselves a facade of righteousness and morality. We will not deal with them— nothing to analyze there. They just bolted and that is the end of our interest; the continuation of what they do after moving away or staying in a detached relationship is material for tabloids. The tabloids, by the way, have done a sensational job on some personalities, some very recent cases, including the one when the husband served divorce papers while his wife was in the hospital.

He may be devastated by this life-altering news, and enter into a state of complete helplessness.

He may rely completely on the advice of his wife's doctor; follow all of their instructions; rely completely on their medical expertise. (This is often the case, since the woman in his life has already emotionally and intellectually put her life in the hands of the doctors she has come to thrust.)

But for a special and dauntless group of men-who refuse to take "no" for an answer; who reject the idea their wife will be ultimately lost; the End is not at hand. They fight the good fight. They challenge the diagnosis of the doctors, and they read and learn every detail of the wife's disease.

There are countless case histories - sacred stories of how husbands have prolonged the lives of their wives.

Case 1: William without a will.

His wife was 56 when she was diagnosed with late stage cervical cancer. At first when William learned the news - as his wife Cora explained it, with tears in his eyes, he leaned back on the sofa, and felt that he was stuck in the eyes with a sharp stick.

"How do we fight this thing?" was his first reaction.

"I have to take several tests," his wife Cora responded.

And it was at that moment that William made a heartfelt decision to put Cora's health totally into the hands of the doctors. He asked no questions. Didn't doubt a moment that his wife's doctors knew precisely what treatment was necessary. Six weeks of radiation, endless weeks of Chemotherapy and countless hours spent in waiting rooms for Cora's visits.

William did not ask the questions whirling through his mind. With all the strength of the love, he bore for his wife, he inwardly raged at the fact that he was helpless to do anything to help.

William sought solace in Scotch. These few drinks a day became a necessary release from sorrow and helplessness.

He sat at her bedside the night Cora finally expired filled with painkillers - her head wrapped in a scarf. William looked at Cora's emaciated face, remembered the luxurious light brown hair that had swirled around her shoulders. All gone now - thanks to the chemotherapy that was meant to kill the cancerous cells that had infested her body.

He held her hand as the last breath eased from her mouth, and he kissed her lips, and dropped his own tears on her gray cheek.

"I could have done something," he said to himself. I could have fought this battle with you". But I did not know how, Cora I did not know how."

To this day William regrets his inability to have taken an active and intelligent part in helping cure his wife's cancer - or at least helping to prolong and ease her life. William has not forgiven himself.

Case 2: Ciro makes himself scarce.

He was a film editor, working in Burbank California; He did not edit movies, but was exceptionally adept when it came to editing 30-second television commercials. Indeed, he was able to take the two hours of film that the commercial director had filmed days earlier, and pick the perfect "takes," slice them apart on his Movieola and splice the pieces together again for maximum effect.

He was married to his craft, devoted to his successful career and was willing to work around the clock to meet any deadline thrown at him.

He also was married to Lois, who was supportive of his career, and a model mother to the couple's teenage male twins.

One evening, after dinner his sons said to him - almost in unison - "something is really disturbing Mom. She will not give us a heads-up on what is happening. Maybe you can get something out of her?"

As Ciro and Lois prepared for bed on that evening, he heard his wife's voice coming from the dressing room as she brushed her hair.

"Ciro I have cancer of the uterus."

Ciro sitting on the edge of the bed, wearing a t -Shirt and Jockey shorts, and leafing through a film trade journal, suddenly brought his chin up and clenched his fists.

"Come out here Lois," he snapped. "Come out here and tell me what's going on."

Lois sat beside her husband at the edge of their bed. Suddenly she slumped back onto the bedspread, and began to wipe away, with the sleeve of her pajamas, the tears that were forming at the corners of her eyes.

"I am so scared, Ciro" she sobbed. "Really scared to death. I wake up at 4 o'clock in the morning in cold sweat, and think about all the pain that I am going to experience - and the pain I am going to cause you and our sons."

Ciro brought his hand to Lois's shoulder, rubbed her back and kissed her cheek. "Don't worry, sweetheart," he murmured," you'll beat this thing. You are strong. You're tough. We can afford to get you the best of care."

As the following weeks turned into months, Ciro found himself spending countless hours with Lois in the waiting rooms of a number of doctors, Inwardly, he began to resent these times; wasted hours that were taking him away from his work. Then came the weeks of radiation and chemotherapy. Again, he sat with Lois, holding her hand, forcing himself to be encouraging.

Finally, one evening, he sat with two sons in the kitchen of their home while Lois was upstairs in their bedroom. "Look," he said, with an edge of anger in his voice, "my business is going to hell. Clients want my personal attention, and I am spending hours and hours with your mother at the doctors during her treatments. You guys are going to have to pitch in. Starting tomorrow, I'll check in with you and mom every day, and I'll be here when you really need me."

And so, it went for the next several weeks, until one day, as Ciro sat in front of his Movieola, editing a series of high-priced commercials for

Coca-Cola, he received a phone call from one of his sons.

"Dad, we went to mom's doctor, this morning," said Dennis. "Mom is terminal. She won't recover from her cancer. The doctor gives her less than six months".

Ciro felt his blood run cold. He sat in front of his Movieola- hearing its raspy whirl. And somewhere in the sound of the machine he felt a sudden detachment to all near and dear in his life. He turned off the machine with an angry flip of the switch. And with that flip of that switch, he emotionally removed himself from any contact with his wife and family.

Ciro knew full well the weakness he held in his heart. A weakness that prevented him from being a loving partner in his wife's death; he could not, in any way, bring himself to visit Lois at the hospice as she passed into another world.

These days, he sits in front of his beloved editing machine, and lost in the harsh rasp of the Movieola, he faces the fact, on a daily basis, that he did not possess the courage to remain at the side of his wife as she battled her cancer.

His sons understood his weakness, and in their own way, promised themselves that they would be stronger men than their father ever was.

Case 3: Benjamin the Brave Heart

Benjamin was the CEO of one of the leading architectural firms in the mid-West.
His future seemed warm and rosy and blessed by God to succeed.

He was in his late 40s, and a big robust, handsome man. The kind of a man that women of all ages would have liked to take to bed.

However, Benjamin was a faithful husband. He detested President Bill Clinton for all his infidelities, and although he was progressive in his political thoughts, he often said, "If you can lie to your wife, you can lie to the rest of the world."

Benjamin's wife who was a heavy smoker was diagnosed with throat cancer. Benjamin who smoked no more than a half dozen cigarettes a day, battled to give up the habit.

Benjamin and Karen had two daughters, who became instantly alarmed when learning about their mother's sickness. Benjamin was a decisive man - always ready to make quick, but thoughtful decisions, a quality that made him invaluable to his clients.

Once he fully grasped the nature and seriousness of his wife's condition, he turned all his formidable power to understand every facet of throat cancer.

He joined Karen on every one of her visits to the doctors; He visited every web site on his computer to increase his knowledge of his wife's cancer. He haunted Barnes& Noble and plucked every book from the shelf that would point him in directions to prolong Karen's life – perhaps to even cure her sickness.

He challenged his wife, doctors; not in an offensive way, but to learn everything they knew. To understand every nuance of throat cancer.

Benjamin concentrated all his intelligence on the use of alternative and complement ways. And soon, Benjamin and Karen began to see results. Karen had lost a considerable amount of her hair, due to radiation and chemotherapy, but soon, her hair began to grow back. Her health improved, the supplemental actions Benjamin took mitigated and complemented all those poisonous treatments she received in the clinic, and blessedly his wife cooperated. The smile returned to her lips. She had beaten her hideous cancer. She had forged a renewed loving bond with her husband. No, it did not happen overnight. No, it wasn't a miracle. It took hard work. Intelligent work on the part of both of them, especially Benjamin.

And there is a warm and rosy spot in his heart at what he achieved. He felt that he had designed the highest building in the world. Perhaps, some day he will do that too.

Neither the author, Sven Sonnenberg, nor the publisher, hold medical degrees and claim no responsibility for particular results of any person. This book is an account of what the author credits helping his own wife, Elizabeth Sonnenberg, live a longer, higher quality life while fighting cancer.

www.ingramcontent.com/pod-product-compliance
Lightning Source LLC
Chambersburg PA
CBHW060557200326
41521CB00007B/598